MULTIPLE SCLEROSIS

QUESTIONS AND ANSWERS

DAVID BARNES

Foreword by
IAN McDONALD

merit
PUBLISHING
INTERNATIONAL

MERIT PUBLISHING INTERNATIONAL

European address:
1st Fl., 35 Winchester Street
Basingstoke, Hampshire
RG21 7EE
England
E-mail: merituk@aol.com

North American address:
8260 NW 49th Manor
Coral Springs, Florida
33067
U.S.A.
E-mail: meritpi@aol.com

Web: www.meritpublishing.com

ISBN 1 873413 86 6

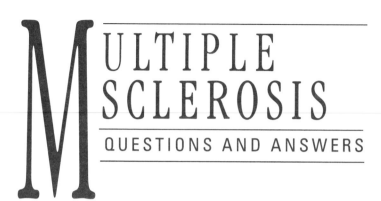

MULTIPLE SCLEROSIS

QUESTIONS AND ANSWERS

DAVID BARNES
Consultant Neurologist, Atkinson Morley's Hospital,
London, England

Foreword by
PROFESSOR IAN McDONALD
Royal College of Physicians, London, England

m*e*rit
PUBLISHING
INTERNATIONAL

MULTIPLE SCLEROSIS

CONTENTS

MULTIPLE SCLEROSIS

MULTIPLE SCLEROSIS

FOREWORD

Exciting developments are taking place in our understanding of Multiple Sclerosis and how it can be treated. In the past decade there have been notable advances in our appreciation of how the brain is damaged, what influences susceptibility to the disease and what causes the irrecoverable disability so common in its later stages.

One consequence of this progress has been the improved symptomatic management and the development of the first treatments, which modify the course of Multiple Sclerosis. They are only partially effective but new strategies are being developed which can be assessed much more quickly and was possible previously. MRI is making an invaluable contribution, as it is to the facilitation of early and accurate diagnosis. The role of these new treatments in different groups of patients is still being defined. As a result, people with Multiple Sclerosis have many questions about the disease and how it will affect them in the future; whether other family members will develop it, whether the form and manifestations of the illness that they have are amenable to treatment, and what is the risk/benefit of treatment.

In this publication, Dr. David Barnes draws on his wide experience of the disease to provide a practical approach to answering these and many other questions. Neurologists, family physicians and general practitioners, residents, informed carers, and people with Multiple Sclerosis will find it invaluable in their day-to-day activities.

Professor Ian McDonald
Royal College of Physicians
London, England

MULTIPLE SCLEROSIS

INTRODUCTION

The prevalence of MS worldwide varies markedly with latitude, race and other factors described later, but particular areas of high prevalence are the northern USA, Western Europe, parts of East Asia, New Zealand, and Southern Australia. In the USA, for example, the prevalence overall is just over 100 per 100,000 of the population, but varies from under 50 in Florida to nearly 200 in some of the northern states.

The specialist, particularly one with an interest in MS, quickly learns that although there are a limited number of useful strategies available to deal with the wide range of clinical problems, such as bladder dysfunction, these strategies can be highly effective.

The real skill lies in integrating these various therapies to the best advantage of the patient. It is certainly the case that most practitioners, with a little effort, can acquire the necessary skills to improve their management of these patients to the point where specialist input is less frequently or urgently required. In many parts of the world where MS has a high prevalence, specialist neurologists are relatively scarce or inaccessible or both.

Family Practitioners and patients perceive this lack of access to specialist input all too clearly and combined with a general feeling of lack of support at times of need, it represents the commonest source of dissatisfaction expressed by patients on a regular basis. In Canada, by contrast there is a highly developed network of MS specialists who meet on a regular basis to update their knowledge at a very high level. They communicate by e-mail and other means to maintain a very high standard of care for their patients who live great distances apart and are much more likely to have access to an interested specialist than in most parts of the world.

In the UK, with an estimated 80,000 diagnosed individuals, multiple sclerosis (MS) is the second commonest cause, after traumatic brain injury, of neurological disability in young adults.

Approximately 1 per 800-1000 of the population is affected and most General Practitioners will have relatively few patients. They cannot be expected to have acquired the expertise needed to deal with the range of problems which might arise in an MS sufferer, and will rightly turn to the specialist for help in managing patients with active disease or significant fixed disability. Furthermore, the clinical manifestations and natural history of the disease are often highly variable and unpredictable.

The MS population, therefore, presents substantial challenges to health care professionals in terms of both quality and quantity of care available. There is no more than one neurologist for every 250,000 of the population overall, and of necessity most time is spent dealing with acute or urgent problems on a day-by-day basis.

It is difficult to see how the overall situation might be improved until the are substantial increases in specialist numbers and resources for patients. In truth, however, the specialist need not be the most important person in the arena, and potential strategies for the development of nurse-led teams of carers will be discussed later in this book.

In summary, from the patient perspective, their main challenges are first to obtain the necessary input at times of need, equating to a feeling of support, and secondly to educate themselves about their disease to a level which provides insight into their disabilities and what can and cannot be done to help.

The aim of this important book, is to provide a brief outline of the nature of MS and how it is likely to affect individuals both short and long-term, a rational approach to its diagnosis, and an overview of symptomatic and other management strategies available to any doctor who cares to find out. The role of the specialist is not to deal with all problems as they arise, but to be quickly available to help in more difficult situations. Also, the specialist should coordinate the overall strategy of services to be provided for his or her MS population, and expand and develop those services as required.

It is hoped that the contents of this book will be of most use to Family and General Practitioners, residents, junior neurologists, interns, medical students and carers with a specific interest, as well as informed patients. More senior colleagues might find themselves dipping at random should it land on their desks, if only to criticize, an enjoyable activity at the best of times; but they might accidentally learn something, in which case I will be well satisfied.

CHAPTER 1

DEFINITION AND HISTORICAL ASPECTS

1.1 What is Multiple Sclerosis?

MS is the commonest of a group of diseases whose pathological hallmarks are inflammation and demyelination. The cause of MS remains elusive, though in recent years, a number of advances have been made, particularly in relation to the contribution of genetic susceptibility and the pathological evolution of lesions over time. Its clinical manifestations are highly variable and somewhat unpredictable, and herein lie the main challenges to effective management. Approximately 85% of sufferers will develop the disease in early adult life in the form of relapsing-remitting MS (RRMS) and after ten years at least half will enter a secondary progressive phase (SPMS) of the illness during which disability is permanent and worsening at a variable rate.

The clinical relapse (or attack) of MS is characteristic and defined as the appearance of new or the worsening of old symptoms and signs lasting at least 24 hours. Relapses are considered separate if they occur more than one month apart. The diagnosis depends heavily on clinical findings of damage to more than one part of the central nervous system (CNS) over time, and will be considered in more detail in Chapter 4. Although MS as a disease is much feared, the prognosis in general is not as poor as commonly thought. Some 5-10% of patients will never develop significant fixed disability (benign MS), and at least a third will remain fully independent when not in relapse.

1.2 What happens at the beginning?

Once the diagnosis has been made, it is crucial that the patient is given time and opportunity to ask questions, and an explanation is given of the nature of the condition and what to do at times of trouble. Initial acceptance of the disease is very difficult for some, and additional problems may arise with partners and other family members who cannot come to terms with what has happened. It is most important that this initial phase is properly managed if long-term problems beyond the purely physical are to be minimized.

Patient support groups are not to everybody's taste, but can offer valuable support to some families, and the relevant National MS Society or Association which exists in most countries, will usually provide helpful material on request. Education is every bit as important as accurate diagnosis at this stage. The next few years will often set the pattern of the disease in any one individual, and the informed specialist should be able to offer some sort of overall prognosis reasonably quickly. It is no longer acceptable either to tell patients that the prognosis is too variable to be predicted usefully, or to give the impression that every problem is MS-related and therefore nothing can be done.

Patients need to know that help is available when required, and that symptomatic treatment will often improve quality of life significantly. Furthermore, for the first time in the history of the disease, we are now entering an exciting period of progress in treatments which beneficially influence the natural history of MS, with both the ß-interferons and glatiramer acetate (formerly known as Copolymer-1) having been shown in well conducted clinical trials to be effective in suppressing disease activity in selected groups of patients.

While there is still no approach to a cure for MS, its path can, now more than ever, be made much smoother because of recent advances in our understanding of MS and the rational development of treatment for symptoms, relapses and disease activity overall. Sympathetic handling of the initial diagnostic and post-diagnostic stages, the provision of adequate education and support and appropriate use of these modern treatments are beginning to make a substantial contribution to reducing the impact overall of this much feared disease.

1.3 Where did the story start?

There are accounts of probable MS dating back to the 14th century, but the history of the disease really begins in the 19th century with the first illustrations and clear clinical descriptions of the disease beginning to appear from 1838. For an authoritative account of the early history of MS the interested reader is referred to Compston (1988).[1] Herein he explains

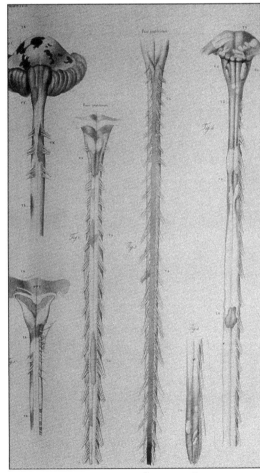

that *Jean Martin Charcot* is generally credited with pulling together the clinical threads of MS, publishing in 1868 clear descriptions of patients whose symptoms began in the mid-1850s; subsequently the disease was ascribed eponymously to him by *Althaus* in 1877. However, the first patients in whom the diagnosis could be made with reasonable certainty were described by *CP d'Angieres Ollivier* as early as 1824, and in the famous diary, of *Auguste D'Esté* which only came to light in 1940. There is a personal account of his own disease which began in 1822 with optic neuritis, and subsequently followed a typical relapsing remitting pattern of neurological activity and eventually substantial fixed disability by the mid 1840s.

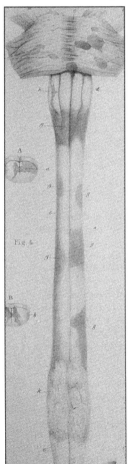

Figure 1:   The first depiction of the lesions of MS (from Carswell 1838)
Figure 1.1: The lesions of MS (from Cruveilhier 1841)

MULTIPLE SCLEROSIS

CHAPTER 2

EPIDEMIOLOGY AND ETIOLOGY

The first depiction of the actual lesions of MS appeared 160 years ago, and it was the Scot, Robert Carswell who produced the first drawings of spinal cord plaques in 1838. This honor might have been bestowed upon the great Jean Cruveilhier, but it seems that he missed the boat by publishing his observations serially, so that while they may have been the first existing drawings, publication only came in 1841, three years after Carswell. By 1875 the disease was becoming well recognized with clear case descriptions appearing, among other places, in the Lancet anonymously from 1873-1875; patients nearly all from Guy's Hospital, London.

Other notable contributions include those of Ramon Cajal who described demyelination and had ideas about its origins, and Dawson who described his "fingers" as radial lines of perivenular demyelination arising from the corpus callosum. This observation is fundamental to our current thinking of the origin of the lesions as a form of venulitis.

From these early descriptions, our understanding of the nature of MS has grown, and it is remarkable how many of the insights of these early scientists have not only stood the test of time, but are revisited as confirmation that our own, sometimes less secure observations may be valid.

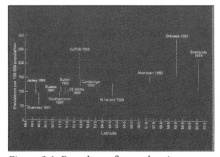

Figure 2.1: Prevalence figure showing North-South gradient of MS

2.1 How common is Multiple Sclerosis?

This question is deceptively simple: the answer is that in some parts of the world it is very common but in others, almost non-existent. As with many diseases, epidemiological studies of MS are beset by technical difficulties and variations in methodology. These studies can tell us where and who MS strikes, and might provide insights into the cause or contributing factors. In general, the commonness of MS varies with latitude, being lowest near the equator, and becoming more common at increasing latitudes both north and south of the equator.

Figures for the USA are as would be expected at any given latitude, being 110-165 in the central states. The explanation for these gradients is unclear.[2] The disease is most common in temperate regions: In the British and Channel Isles, the prevalence (per 105 of the population) ranges from 87-113 in Jersey and Guernsey, through 115 in south-east England, 122 in north-west England, to 158 in southern Scotland and 178 in the Highlands. In the southern hemisphere, northern New Zealand has a prevalence of 22-24, middle 72 and the south island 77-79. Similarly in northern Australia it is 11-18, further south 33-38, and in Hobart, 74.

2.2 Where and who does Multiple Sclerosis strike?

Migration studies have provided tantalizing clues of environmental influence in the development of MS. In the 1950s, Dean showed that in South Africa, the age-adjusted frequency of MS was highest in immigrants from Europe, intermediate in South African English and low in Afrikaaners.[3] The absolute absence of MS in black Africans was also confirmed. Interestingly, among the English-speaking whites, those coming from Northern Europe as adults brought with them the frequency of their country of origin, whereas those emigrating below the age of 15 showed the rate of their adopted country. Similarly in the UK, immigrants arriving as children, regardless of racial origin, seem to acquire the rate of their new home. These data give a clear indication that there is some environmental trigger which allows the expression of the disease in young people, perhaps through a genetic or immunological susceptibility which no longer operates in mature adults.

Such data, however, are not without limitations: migrants are not necessarily representative of the general population; the host country may place restrictions with health status implications on

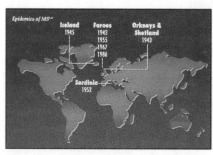

Figure 2.2: Epidemics of MS

immigrants; and immigrants may not necessarily experience the same
environmental conditions as the indigenous population by reasons of uneven
distribution, forming their own communities and leading their own lifestyles
rather than fully integrating. Nevertheless, there are enough studies of this type
to draw general conclusions about the impact of migration at differing ages on
the commonness of MS.

Further evidence for environmental factors at work comes from studies of
apparent outbreaks of the disease. Perhaps the best-documented
"epidemic" occurred in the Faroe Islands.[4] A search for cases with onset
before the Second World War revealed no patients whose disease began
before 1943. Thereafter, 16 cases were identified with onset from 1943 and

1949 and a further 16 to 1973. It
is difficult to avoid the
conclusion that some
environmental factor was
introduced to the Faroes after
1943 which caused the disease
to appear. The most popular
explanation suggests that it was
the occupation of the island
from 1940-1945 by British troops
that was responsible. While some

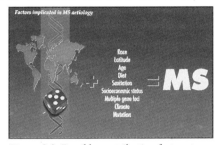

Figure 2.3: Possible contributing factors to
the development of MS in an individual

remain unconvinced, citing such criticisms as accuracy of diagnosis, the
close temporal and spatial relationship between the occupation and case
development is persuasive to most. Whether this and other similar
"epidemics" can be taken as conclusive evidence that MS is a transmissible
disease, or whether some other mechanism(s) are responsible remains
unclear.

These, and other epidemiological clues have been extremely valuable as
indicators of the factors which determine the prevalence of MS in any
particular part of the world. Within the limitations of such surveys, there
appears no doubt that a particular environment contains elements, which
can stimulate the development of MS in a susceptible individual.

2.3 What else might contribute to the onset of Multiple Sclerosis?

There are a large number of other factors, in addition to those discussed
already, which seem to influence the commonness of MS in general, and
the risk to any one individual in particular. All studies agree that MS is

commoner in women than men in a ratio of about 2:1. In teenagers the ratio is nearer 3:1, and over 45 it is 2.4:1.

Among a racially mixed indigenous population such as the USA, racial origin is clearly important: if white males are taken as 1, black males have a relative risk of 0.43 and Asians 0.22. Other potential culprits with greater or lesser scientific validity include diet and nutrition, hygiene and sanitation, and "urbanization": in general the higher the standards the higher the apparent risk!.

2.4 If it's in the family, will I get Multiple Sclerosis?

The short answer is probably not. There is no doubt that genetic factors play a part in the development of MS by conferring varying degrees of individual susceptibility. MS has a familial recurrence rate of about 15% overall. The Canadian study of familial MS took a baseline risk of 0.2% and showed a risk of 3% in first degree relatives, and 1% in second degree relatives. More specifically, in the UK the risk is increased as follows: sister, 4.4%; brother, 3.2%; parent, 2.1%; child, 1.8%; all first and second degree relatives, 2.8 and 1% respectively.[5] Where both parents have MS, the risk to offspring is significantly higher, with an age-adjusted rate about ten times that of children with only one affected parent, so approaching 20%.

Twin studies are a valuable tool for exploring the genetic component of risk for any disease with multifactorial causation: if there is observed difference between pairs of identical and non-identical twins, then, assuming the environment of both types to be the same at the relevant stage of life, the difference must be due to genetic factors. There are practical problems with twins studies, such as ascertainment, and a tendency to over-representation of females and identical twin pairs, but assuming these problems are identified and controlled for, the outcome can provide highly valuable information.

In MS, all studies except one from France show similar results. For identical twins the concordance rate is 25-30%, whereas for non-identical twins it is approximately the same as ordinary siblings at 3% genetic mechanisms (probably several in any one person), and possibly time-dependent factors such as current immune status and other infection. One thing is certain. We do not know the cause of MS, and so far no one has come close.

CHAPTER 3

THE PATHOLOGICAL EVOLUTION OF THE LESION

3.1 What happens in the acute lesion of Multiple Sclerosis?

A simple understanding of the pathological processes which characterize the lesion of MS at different times in its development is fundamental to the management of the disease. The knowledge, for example that in acute optic neuritis, the severity of the pain, visual impairment and loss of amplitude of the visual evoked potential correlates with the degree of active inflammation in the nerve helps us to decide whether the potential benefits of high dose steroids might outweigh the potential risks. The demonstrable correlation between certain symptoms and pathological processes adds to our ability to explain to our patients what is happening and the rationale for treatment offered.

Magnetic resonance imaging (MRI) studies have shown that one of the first events in the evolution of a new lesion in MS in breach of the blood-brain barrier (BBB). This process is concentrated on small veins as originally observed by Dawson. In effect, therefore, MS can be considered as a form of vasculitis, the process being confined to the CNS including the retina. The sites of predilection of this process for symptomatic lesions, namely the optic nerve, brainstem and cervical spinal cord remains unexplained.

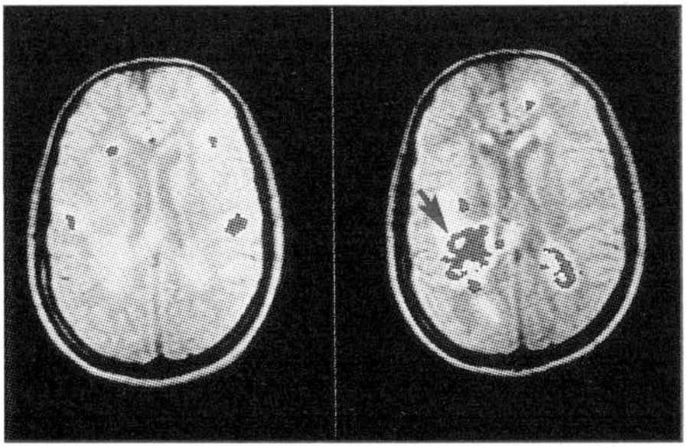

Figure 3.1:T_1-weighted MRI of brain in MS. Areas of BBB damage shown as enhancement in active MS (arrowed)

Our understanding of the process initiating the inflammation of cerebral veins in MS has become more complete in the last decade with the discovery and characterization of soluble inflammatory mediators known as cytokines, and the ways in which the influence the behavior of immune-competent cells and vascular endothelium. The initiating factor, possibly the cause of MS remains speculative. In the animal model of experimental allergic encephalomyelitis, similar processes can be stimulated by components of myelin or the introduction of suitably primed lymphocytes. Although anti-myelin antibodies can be identified in the serum of patients with MS, they may also be present in control subjects, and do not clearly correlate with disease activity. Furthermore, their presence does not prove that they are primary elements in the inflammatory cascade.

By whatever mechanism, T-lymphocytes in particular are specifically targeted against the vascular wall, and by secreting cytokines recruit other cells including macrophages. Adhesion molecules and their receptor molecules expressed on the lymphocyte and endothelial cell allow the former to adhere to the vessel wall, following which they punch a hole through the endothelium, or occasionally through the intercellular space, pass through the basement membrane, and so enter the CNS.

Once inside these cells are able to recruit non-specifically microglia and other lymphocytes to produce a perivascular inflammatory lesion. Tissue damage results from release of molecules such as complement forming

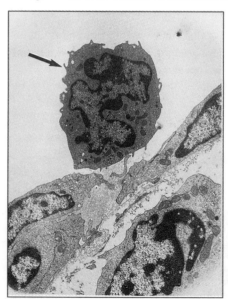

membrane attack complexes and cytokines such as TNF which is capable of injuring myelin following which macrophages ingest the resulting myelin fragments.

The inflammatory phase may last only a few days, or may persist for a month, and the end result will depend on the intensity and duration of the attack. Functionally, the involved region is impaired, and depending upon its location may, or more likely will not produce a clinical deficit. There is recent evidence to indicate that the release of nitric oxide within acutely

Figure 3.2: Lymphocyte (arrow) attaching to CNS vascular endothelial cell junction

inflamed lesions may cause further functional and structural injury to the tissues. This release is dependent on activation of axons within the lesion. Structurally this inflammatory phase is associated with the development of vasogenic edema following BBB breakdown, which may extend a considerable distance from the center of the lesion. With repair of the BBB, the edema resolves, usually over a few weeks, leaving a residual scar.

3.2 What happens in the older lesion?

Following resolution of the inflammation phase of the lesion, there is potential for repair. Contrary to traditional belief, the CNS of the adult human does contain cells capable of remyelinating denuded axons. Such repair, unfortunately, is not complete, though some degree of functional recovery is possible. In the early stages of the disease, when recovery from relapses is the norm, demyelination is not likely to be a prominent factor, and it is the inflammation itself, which causes the symptoms. As the disease progresses, however, repeated attacks lead to permanent structural injury, though even then, the CNS fights, compensating by modifying sodium channel configuration to optimize conduction in demyelinated segments of the axon. Finally, however, the struggle is lost as these repair and compensatory mechanisms are overwhelmed, and fixed functional deficits arise.

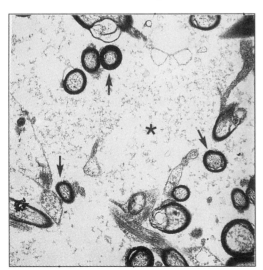

Figure 3.3: Chronic "open" lesion of MS. Few remaining axons (arrowed) float in vastly expanded extracellular space (*)

The precise mechanism(s) whereby permanent or fixed clinical disability appears is not clear, but the biggest contributor to this dreaded outcome is probably axonal loss, though several mechanisms may contribute. The end result is the chronic MS plaque, a region of denuded axons surrounded by intense gliosis due to astrocyte proliferation which may impair function further.

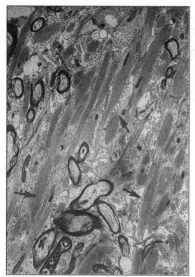

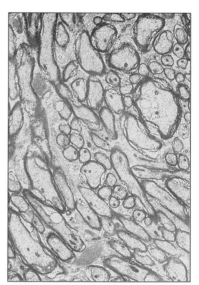

Figure 3.4a: Chrome "closed" version of MS. Space left by axonal loss filled with astrocytic processes (arrowed) no extracellular space apparent

Figure 3.4b: Normal-appearance white matter showing preservation of axons for comparison with Figure 3.4a

Electron microscopy of these lesions shows a range of appearances from "closed" regions where axons, though demyelinated, are largely retained and may have residual function, through to "open" regions where the extracellular space occupies large volumes of the tissue within which a few denuded axons swing uselessly among astrocyte processes. There can be no recovery from this endpoint.

It is entirely unclear why some individuals with MS run a benign course and others a much more malignant one. Perhaps the former have a CNS with a greater capacity for recovery, or perhaps we are dealing with several diseases all called multiple sclerosis. Similarly, the typical relapsing-remitting form of the disease may or may not evolve into a chronically progressive phase, and there appear to be no reliable indicators to predict this outcome. The onset of a

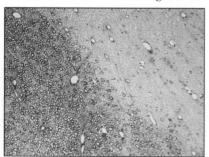

Figure 3.5: Interface between normally myelinated and demyelinated white matter

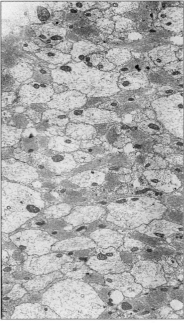

Figure 3.5a: "Open" chrome vesion of MS

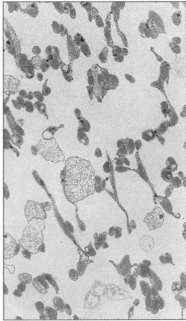

Figure 3.5b: "Closed" chrome vesion of MS

progressive phase seems to indicate that the pathological process, hitherto periodic, now has enough momentum of its own to persist without outside help from agents such as infections and hormonal changes known to increase the risk of relapse. Possibly at this stage, the BBB, repetitively breached in the past, no longer has the capacity to repair itself, allowing a continuing low-grade inflammation process to eat away the tissue, a hypothesis which would fit the observation that it is existing deficit that progresses, new deficits appearing well into the progressive phase, for example optic neuritis for the first time, being relatively uncommon.

The basic science which has allowed these insights into the natural pathological history of MS has gathered considerable momentum in the last ten years, and is beginning to reap dividends in the form of several putative treatments to influence the natural history of the disease itself. Some, like IFN-b have become established if not universally accepted treatment albeit with substantial limitations; others like linamide, showed even more promise but failed because of unforeseen side effects; yet others like anti-lymphocyte globulin appear simply not to work. They all have in common the fact that their development was based on rational observation, and it should not be too long before the right substance or combination of substances finally make a major impact on this pathological chain of events. Progress has been made also in studying the process of remyelination, and its artificial promotion, though as yet success of a meaningful nature remains elusive.

CHAPTER 4

THE DIAGNOSIS OF MULTIPLE SCLEROSIS

4.1 What are the principles involved in making a diagnosis?

The most important principle to consider when diagnosing MS is whether the person fulfils the diagnostic criteria on clinical grounds. There is, as yet, no diagnostic test for the disease. While laboratory investigations, including evoked potentials, lumbar puncture and MRI, may be valuable adjuncts to diagnosis, it is the clinical evaluation which remains of paramount importance. It is not possible to diagnose definite MS without clear evidence of damage to the CNS in more than one site, disseminated in time, and without an adequate alternative explanation. That having been said, we are inevitably relying more heavily on MRI in particular for improving diagnostic precision both for confirmation and exclusion of other possible diagnoses.

The most widely used diagnostic criteria are those of Poser (1983).[7] These criteria are largely a matter of common sense and are helpful in everyday clinical practice. More importantly, they were intended to provide a formal basis upon which the diagnosis could be classified for research purposes. It should be recognized, however, that despite their merits such criteria are only an adjunct to accurate diagnosis: they take no account of other possible causes of the same clinical presentation and do not define the small but important primary progressive category of patients (see Chapter 6).

From these criteria it can be seen that, it is possible to make a definite diagnosis after only one relapse provided oligoclonal bands (OCB) are present in the cerebrospinal fluid (CSF). In clinical practice, however, as emphasized above, it would generally be considered preferable to establish clinically that the disease is disseminated in both time and space before imparting a definite diagnosis. The demonstration of dissemination in time is generally straightforward, and requires only that the interval between attacks was more than one month.

Category	Minimum number of:		Paraclinical Evidence	Oligoclonal Bands
	Relapses	Deficits		
Clinically definite	2	2		
	2	1 and	1	
Clinically probable	2	1		
	1	2		
	1	1 and	1	
Lab-supported definite	2	1 or	1*	+
	1	2		+
Lab-supported probable	1	1 and	1	+
	2			+

Table 4.1   Poser criteria for the diagnosis of MS.

* Progression of MRI abnormalities over time also constitutes paraclinical evidence for diagnosis of laboratory-supported definite MS.

Sometimes the first attack may have been too long ago to allow clear characterization, in which case it cannot be used, strictly speaking, to make the diagnosis. It is important to realize that an attack should be associated with documented neurological deficits to be of certain value. A vague memory of a week of double vision for which medical advice was not sought is insufficient, but a similar attack clearly documented by a reliable examiner can be considered diagnostically valid. More usually the diagnosis will be seriously considered on the basis of recent events, where the situation is simpler. Care is still required, however, in the interpretation of the patient's deficits in terms of anatomical localization. To establish dissemination in space takes more clinical skill. For example, an episode of sensory disturbance down one side followed by an episode of vertigo and facial numbness could be interpreted as separate locations or as two brainstem attacks at very much the same site. Care is required in this type of situation, and it is preferable to err on the side of caution until there is more certain spatial dissemination of disease. An attack of unilateral visual loss followed by an attack of double vision, on the other hand, can only be caused by lesions in first the optic nerve, and then the brainstem. Now there is no uncertainty, and provided the episodes were clearly documented, occurred more than one month apart, and no better explanation is forthcoming, then the diagnosis is clinically definite MS.

The physical examination is of great importance to the diagnostic process. As well as establishing the signs referable to any current symptoms, a skilled examiner may well be able to elicit abnormalities, which go a long way towards proving dissemination of the disease process in space. Although a thorough approach will often be rewarded, most important is careful examination of the eyes: a previous attack of optic neuritis may well declare itself as a pale or atrophic optic disc associated with a relative afferent pupillary defect on the swinging light test and impaired color vision, if not central acuity. A brainstem attack may well leave behind it an abnormality of eye movements, most characteristically an internuclear ophthalmoplegia (as often as not bilateral), but most commonly dysmetria of pursuit or some form of sustained nystagmus.

In summary, the diagnosis of MS is primarily clinical and depends upon the reliable demonstration of damage to the CNS which is disseminated in both time and space, and for which there is no better explanation. Laboratory investigation is mainly aimed at excluding alternative diagnoses, but in specific circumstances can be used as evidence in favor of MS and can allow a diagnosis of definite MS to be made if it is only probable on clinical grounds by demonstrating lesions additional to those clinically apparent. While, to the practicing clinician, these considerations may appear somewhat pedantic, diagnostic precision is important at all times. Over the years, any busy neurologist will encounter numerous unfortunate examples of people carrying the diagnosis, planning their lives accordingly, but in whom the diagnosis of MS is far from clear.

4.2 Which investigations might be helpful?

From the Poser criteria it can be seen that paraclinical evidence of CNS damage can upgrade the diagnosis from clinically probable to clinically definite MS after two attacks if there is only clinical evidence (abnormal neurological examination) of one. Clearly such evidence must show a lesion other than the one clinically apparent to establish dissemination in space. Nowadays, such paraclinical evidence usually comes from MRI and will be discussed in detail below, but evoked potentials still have a role to play.

There are three types of evoked potential in common use following on from the work of Halliday and McDonald, there are three types of evoked potential in common use, in establishing the characteristic changes of the visual evoked potential (VEP) in optic neuritis.[8] In principle evoked potentials are quantifiable electrical responses to a specific stimulus applied to a neurological system of interest. VEP may be obtained from the visual cortex following stimulation by pattern-reversal or flash. Somatosensory evoked potentials (SEP) are similar responses recorded from the sensory cortex following a contralateral electrical stimulus of a peripheral nerve, usually on the hand or foot, and brainstem auditory evoked potentials (BSAEP) can be recorded following aural stimulation.

The VEP is a particularly useful tool for demonstrating lesions of the optic nerve of all kinds. In relation to MS, the relevant syndrome is optic neuritis, in which the nerve becomes inflamed and showed the same pathological evolution as described in Chapter 3. The VEP is abnormal from one or both eyes in over 75% of patients with clinically definite MS. In the very early phase of optic neuritis, conduction within the nerve may be blocked and the amplitude of the VEP falls correspondingly, but the more typical finding, reflecting demyelination and therefore slowing of conduction in the optic nerve, is a delay in the response from the affected eye.

An example of how such an abnormality might be diagnostically useful would be a patient presenting with an isolated brainstem syndrome who has a delayed VEP from one eye. According to the Poser criteria, this situation allows a diagnosis of clinically probable MS, and if there is a clear history of another relapse in the past, even without a clinical correlate, the diagnosis can be upgrade to clinically definite MS.

	Evoked potentials		
	VEP	SSEP	BAEP
Specificity for MS	✗	✗	✗
Invasive	✗	✗	✗
Suitable for any patient	✔	✔	✔
Result in CDMS patients	75-97% (+ve)	≤96% (+ve)	67% (+ve)
Detects clinically silent lesions	✔	✔	✔
Pinpoints lesions associated with particular symptoms	✔	✗	✗
Useful in early diagnosis	✔/✗	✔/✗	✔/✗
Gives evidence of dissemination of lesions in space	✔	✔	✔
Gives evidence of dissemination of lesions in time	✗	✗	✗

✔ = yes, ✗ = no, ✔/✗ = uncertain, +ve = positive

Figure 4.1: The usefulness of evoked potentials in the diagnosis of MS

The same principle applies to the SEP and BSAEP though much more care is required in their interpretation as they may be affected by a wide range of conditions, or be abnormal due to the current episode, in which case dissemination is space remains unproven. The SEP has been reported as abnormal in over 90% of patients with established MS, but in the initial evaluation they are of less help because of low specificity. The BSAEP is abnormal in about two-thirds of patients.

In practice, while the VEP is still commonly used the other evoked potentials are now of less value in this context, though both can be in other clinical settings; ENT surgeons in particular make frequent use of the BSAEP, and the SEP can contribute to the evaluation of patients with predominantly sensory problems other than MS.

4.3 What other tests might be needed?

The differential diagnosis of MS will be considered in detail in Chapter 6, and the role of MRI in Chapter 5. Other laboratory tests in relation to the diagnostic process are generally required to exclude other possible causes of the patient's symptoms. A full hematological and biochemical screen, ESR, and autoimmune profile should be performed on all patients. Serological tests for syphilis, vitamin B_{12}, folate and protein electrophoresis may also be appropriate. In some patients, the origin of neurological symptoms may be so obscure that more extensive investigations are required. For example, both peripheral (EMG and nerve conduction studies) and central neurophysiology (SEP and central motor conduction times) may assist in unraveling complicated neurological symptomatology.

The role of lumbar puncture is to some extent, a matter of personal preference among doctors. Some prefer to examine the CSF in all patients with possible MS, others feel there is no place for this test in the routine work up. Again the Poser criteria have something to say: the categories of laboratory supported probable and definite MS are somewhat artificial in that they depend upon the presence of OCB in the CSF which merely reflect non-specifically an immune response in the CNS. They cannot contribute to the demonstration of dissemination nor are they specific for MS.

Currently, common practice is to reserve lumbar puncture for those relatively few patients in whom the diagnosis is unclear, but the evidence supports an immunological or inflammatory process as the possible cause. In these circumstances, the finding of OCB is helpful in terms of

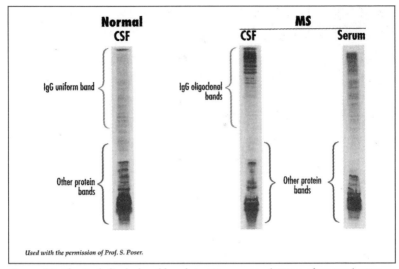

Used with the permission of Prof. S. Poser.

Figure 4.2: Identical oligoloclonal bands in MS serum and CSF confirm production within the CNS

establishing an immunological or inflammatory etiology for the complaint which may or may not be MS, and for management, as it becomes likely that some form of immunosuppressant therapy may benefit the patient. If, however, a patient has clinically probable disease, it would not be appropriate to consider performing a lumbar puncture just to change the diagnostic category to laboratory-supported definite MS, which, as noted above, is somewhat artificial, inexplicable to the patient, and does not change management. All doctors no doubt have their own views, but this approach spares many patients an unpleasant experience with potential complications, and reserves the use of lumbar puncture for a relatively small number of patients whose management is likely to be influenced by the results.

CHAPTER 5

THE ROLE OF MRI IN MULTIPLE SCLEROSIS

5.1 How does MRI work?

Magnetic resonance has been a valuable tool for chemical analysis for most of this century, but the remarkably conceptual leap taken by an equally remarkable coincidence at about the same time by Damadian and Lauturbur in the mid-1970s led to its fundamental properties being turned to the field of medical imaging. This leap was akin to pronouncing the electric juicer to be the future of human transport!. The basic principle of MRI is that certain nuclei, most notably for our purposes the proton, exhibit a property whereby, when aligned in a static magnetic field they can be excited by radiofrequency (RF) pulses and, as they return to the equilibrium state, emit energy at a specific frequency which can be measured.

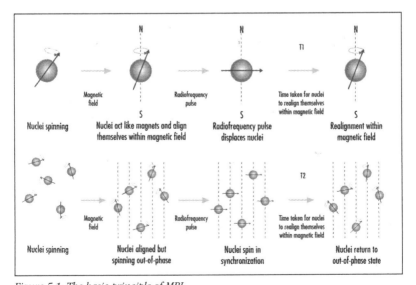

Figure 5.1: The basic principle of MRI

MULTIPLE SCLEROSIS

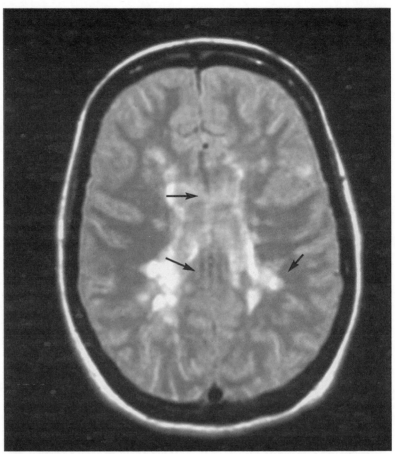

Figure 5.2a: A typical T₂- weighted brain MRI in MS. Periventricular lesions appear as high signal areas (arrowed). Transverse view

In MRI, spatial information can be obtained by superimposing magnetic gradients on the static field which create a similar gradient in the frequencies emitted by relaxing nuclei following excitation. It is the use of such gradients that is the key to MRI. Since the overwhelming majority of protons in biological tissues are contained within water molecules, in its simplest sense, an MR image is a map of tissue water. Variations in the quantity and physical properties of tissue water form the basis of image contrast and define the superb quality of modern MRI. There are several other potential sources of contrast between tissues in MRI, prominent among which are the longitudinal and transverse

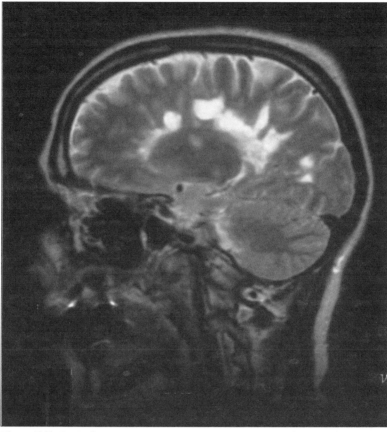

Figure 5.2b: Sagittal view

relaxation times, T_1 and T_2 respectively. These two times describe the rate at which the protons relax back to their resting state after their perturbation by the RF pulse. The imaging parameters can be chosen to optimize the tissue contrast provided by variations between tissues in proton density, T_1 and T_2.

Most disease states, including MS cause changes in the content and properties of tissue water, and therefore are sensitively detected by MRI. Early in the development of MRI it became clear that here, for the first time, was an imaging modality which could not only detect the lesions of MS with great sensitivity, but was also potential free from the types of artifact which degrade traditional CT scanning in certain critical parts of the CNS such as the posterior fossa.

MULTIPLE SCLEROSIS

5.2 What does MRI show in established MS?

Following the initial discovery of its vast potential in a wide range of medical conditions, both neurological and non-neurological, MRI has now developed to the level, not only of providing the best available surrogate for disease activity available in MS, but also to a degree which allows considerable insight to be gained into the fundamental pathological processes at work throughout the evolution of the MS lesion. Of the basic MRI techniques, those which emphasize differences in the T_2 of tissues (T_2-weighted or T_2W sequences) are the most sensitive to the established MS lesion. More recently, a newer technique called FLAIR (FLuid Attenuated Inversion Recovery) has entered routine scanning practice and is even more sensitive than standard T_2W images.

More than 90% of patients with clinically definite MS will have lesions in the brain demonstrable by MRI, most typically in a periventricular distribution, but any part of the neuraxis including the optic nerves can be imaged and may be involved. It must be emphasized, however, than the changes seem on MRI, although sensitive, cannot be considered specific to MS, and may be mimicked by a large number of other neurological diseases including cerebrovascular and vasculitic conditions, sarcoidosis, and leucodystrophies.[9]

5.3 What can MRI tell us about the pathology of MS?

Not least of the developments in MRI techniques has been the introduction of a contrast agent, gadolinium-DTPA (Gd), which allows direct visualization of damage to the BBB. It will be remembered from pathological studies, that the first identifiable event in the evolution of the MS lesion is inflammation, and it is now known that at this stage, Gd enhancement can be seen in most new lesions and is a reliable indicator of the initial inflammatory phase, usually lasting two-six weeks. Recent MRI work suggests, interestingly, that even earlier events can be

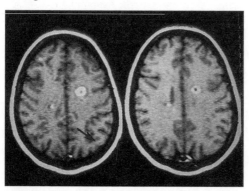

Figure 5.3: Gd-enhanced brain MRI showing areas of BBB leakage in active MS (arrowed)

detected in the normal-appearing white matter prior to the appearance of Gd enhancement.

Subsequently, as edema develops, the volume of Gd enhancement increases as the contrast spreads within the expanded extracellular space. This phase usually reaches its maximum about four weeks after onset, following which repair to the BBB allows absorption and dispersal of the edema fluid, and the volume of the lesion on T₂W images shrinks correspondingly. Ultimately, a residual MRI-visible lesion is left of similar size to the original inflammatory volume. Most new MS lesions go through this cycle, and occasionally may completely disappear, indicating perhaps a capacity for repair or simply minimal damage beyond the resolution of the scanner.

It has already been noted that the end result of the process is a gliotic scar with variable amount of axonal loss. As most chronic MS plaques are visible on T₂W images, the implication is that some degree of axonal loss with expansion of the extracellular space, hence irreversible loss of function, is the rule rather than the exception.

That there is a correlation between what is seen on MRI and what is happening pathologically and clinically has been most clearly established in optic neuritis. The typical attack consists of the onset of pain behind the affected eye, particularly on eye movement. This phase is followed by a progressive though variable loss of acuity, particularly centrally in the affected eye. Subsequently the pain subsides, and, usually some weeks later, acuity returns to normal or near normal in most cases. The initial painful phase correlates consistently with Gd enhancement in the affected nerve indicating that it is actively inflamed: the VEP may drop in amplitude at the same time. The resolution of pain, as might be expected correlates with diminution of enhancement. Finally after the attack subsides, the residual slowing of the VEP, indicating demyelination can sometimes be seen as an asymmetry in the size of the optic nerves on MRI.

In summary, by combining various MRI techniques, all stages of the pathological evolution of the MS lesion can be followed and characterized. Some very small but clinically eloquent lesions may. however, not be seen on imaging, presumably because they are beyond the resolution of standard scanning techniques. This observation is not uncommon with brainstem and spinal cord syndromes in particular. Nevertheless, MRI has now emerged as the most sensitive and valuable modality available for identifying and evaluating the pathological process in MS.

MULTIPLE SCLEROSIS

Newer MR techniques are emerging constantly: for example, a technique called magnetization transfer imaging seems to be able to quantify tissue loss, and MR spectroscopy is also enjoying some popularity as a means of measuring axonal density and loss, and detecting myelin breakdown. Even more research oriented techniques such as magnetization decay curve analysis and others can provide even deeper insights into issue changes accompanying the evolution at the pathological level of this fascinating disease.

It is likely that within a decade, MRI will have taken several further important steps in this area: the introduction of magnetization transfer imaging showing the loss of brain tissue, and spectroscopy, the change in the relative contribution of tissue components, are two good examples.

5.4 How can MRI help with diagnosis?

T_2W or FLAIR MRI will show asymptomatic lesions in over 98% of clinically definite,[10] and over 70% of clinically probable cases. It is true to say that MRI is now the most valuable tool available for confirming the diagnosis of MS and for excluding other possible causes of the patient's problems. It will be remembered from Chapter 4 that the diagnosis of MS remains primarily clinical as detailed in the Poser criteria. A single MRI study may provide paraclinical evidence of spatial dissemination and is more sensitive than other methods like evoked potentials, mainly because it can examine much larger volumes of the nervous system; it is less sensitive than, for example, VEP for the optic nerve alone, but unlike VEP will demonstrate lesions anywhere in the brain or spinal cord if relevant. It has also been noted than while MRI is very sensitive to CNS damage in MS, the appearances are in no way specific and clinical interpretation of the whole picture is required.

Referring to Table 4.1, MRI can upgrade a diagnosis of clinically probably to clinically definite MS, usually by showing asymptomatic deep white matter lesions as paraclinical evidence of dissemination in space. Furthermore, in practical terms, the diagnosis can be considered definite in the situation where after only one attack and with clinical evidence of a single lesion serial MRI is positive and show other lesions developing over time. In practice, very few if any patients will not go on to clinically definite MS in these circumstances, and it might be appropriate to label such patients "MRI-supported definite MS" since dissemination in time and space has been proven. It should be noted that such lesion development will not necessarily be associated with further clinical attacks in the first year or two, as the majority of new MRI activity is asymptomatic.

The usual site of MRI positivity is in the periventricular deep white matter (PVWM); it is unusual for such lesions to be absent in the presence of lesions elsewhere, and such a finding might raise some doubt about the diagnosis. The appearance of the PVWM is generally uneven or beaded, and in coronal section the corpus callosum looks to be "on fire". If the white matter change is smooth and even, the cause is more likely to be vascular disease, and if the lesions are predominantly distributed in the peripheral white matter, near the cortico-medullary junction, the a vasculitic process should be suspected.

In addition to the PVWM, lesions in MS are most commonly found in other parts of cerebral white matter (93%), brainstem (66%) and cerebellum (57%). The cortex (13%) itself and basal ganglia (8%) may be involved, reflecting the pathological observation of at least 5% of lesions in MS brains being confined to grey matter, though such lesions are usually very small and beyond the resolution of the imager. The recent introduction of FLAIR, a new imaging sequence, has increased the overall sensitivity of MRI to MS lesions in some parts of the brain, and is a technique complementary to the traditional T_2W sequences.

Overall MRI has become the most useful technique for demonstrating dissemination of disease in space, and with serial imaging, in time, as an adjunct to the clinical diagnosis of MS, as well as for research and as a marker of disease activity in treatment trials. With further advances it is predictable that formal diagnostic criteria will include categories based on MRI findings to replace the unhelpful existing laboratory-supported category.

5.5 Can an MRI scan help prognostication in clinically isolated syndromes?

Several useful studies have provided data concerning the value of the MRI in determining the likelihood of the person who has suffered an isolated syndrome suggestive of MS going on to develop the disease. Morrissey et al (1993) performed MRI of the brain on such patients with either optic neuritis, or a brainstem or spinal cord syndrome.[11] They found that if the brain MRI was abnormal at presentation, there was a higher risk of developing MS in the next five years than if it was normal (see Table 5.1). Furthermore the risk for fixed disability at five years was also increased.

Types of Isolated Clinical Attack	MRI Abnormal	MRI Normal
Number of Patients	57	32
Progression to MS: All cases	72%	6%
Optic Neuritis	82%	6%
Brainstem Syndrome	67%	0%
Spinal Cord Syndrome	59%	9%

Table 5.1 The risk of developing MS at five years in clinically isolated syndromes *(From Morrissey et al.)[11]*

Types of Isolated Clinical Attack	MRI Abnormal	MRI Normal
Number of Patients	108	54
Progression to MS: All Cases	83%	11%
Optic Neuritis	89%	7%
Brainstem syndrome	91%	0%
Spinal Cord syndrome	67%	25%

Table 5.2 The risk of developing MS at ten years in clinically isolated syndromes *(From O'Riordan et al.)[12]*

The same group of patients formed part of a study of ten year prognosis following presentation with an isolated syndrome published by O'Riordan et al. in 1998 (Table 5.2). From these data, it can be seen that there is a nearly 90% change of developing MS some time in the ten years after optic neuritis if the brain MRI is abnormal at presentation. Furthermore there is also a relationship between the number of lesions visible on the initial MRI and the subsequent prognosis: a single lesion confers a 33% risk whereas three or more confer a greater than 85% chance of MS ten years down the line. In general, the more lesions seen on the original scan, the worse the prognosis overall for both the development of MS and for disability in the next decade.

These data have important implications for our patients with clinically isolated syndromes. It becomes something of a moral and ethical issue whether MS should be mentioned at all after such an attack. Some patients (and experience suggests that it is a substantial proportion) will indicate that they, suspected the diagnosis of MS if it has been mentioned explicitly. In some circumstances, it may be clinically appropriate to carry out a brain MRI to improve prognostication: factors to be considered include the certainty of the clinical diagnosis. For example, in the patient with a spinal lesion that could be inflammatory or could be a tumor, the simplest measure may be to do a brain MRI which, if abnormal, strongly favors an inflammatory cause.

Sometimes patients' wishes need to be considered. The well informed individual will often raise the issue spontaneously, and here it may appropriate to discuss the role of MRI, and to stress that, although it does not necessarily allow a definite diagnosis to be made, it will allow the provision a realistic percentage risk at that stage - time is always the best diagnostic test, and the general experience is that most patients prefer to wait and see what happens. The situation would (and hopefully will) be different if treatment becomes available that would improve the long-term prognosis for those at risk if given early. There are, for instance, trials underway of the use of IFN-b in clinically isolated syndromes, though of necessity these trials will be of long duration, and the answers will not become available within the foreseeable future.

At present, therefore, it is not universal policy routinely to perform brain MRI on patients who have had a single attack consistent with demyelination, for example, optic neuritis, and in whom the nature of the attack is not in doubt. If the patient specifically requests it, then one should be prepared to agree so long as they understand the precise implications of the findings, and that as things stand, there is no likelihood of any useful action being taken on the basis of the findings.

5.6 How good is MRI in different parts of the CNS?

MRI has almost completely replaced myelography in the investigation of patients with both acute and chronic progressive spinal cord lesions. Apart from the obvious practical advantages, it demonstrates the substance of the cord and surrounding soft tissues which are invisible to myelograms. Modern imaging hardware (multi-array coils) enable the entire cord to be images in great detail at one sitting (or, more accurately, lying). Even the

MULTIPLE SCLEROSIS

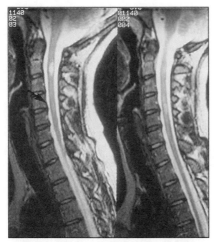

Figure 5.4: Sagittal MRI of spinal cord in the neck. Largest lesion shown by arrow

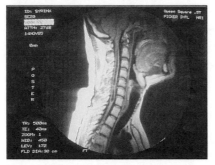

Figure 5.5: Sagittal MRI of neck showing syringomyelia as the cause of symptoms in patient thought to have MS

thoracic spinal cord is now accessible to MRI, where hitherto this region was difficult to image, and the images difficult to interpret because of artifact and poor signal-to noise in the images.

In the context of MS, it is perhaps most useful in excluding other possible causes for the presentation, particularly in primary progressive MS (PPMS: see Chapter 6). This form of MS most commonly presents with a slowly progressive spinal cord syndrome, and it is imperative to exclude compressive and other structural cause as being responsible. Some years ago, the MRI appearances of PPMS were investigated, patients being recruited from specialist centers around the UK. It was, perhaps, surprising that the hit rate for pathology other than MS was so high!

Syringomyelia figured prominently, as did thoracic discs and meningiomas, and herein lies the real value of spinal MRI. It is sensitive to all pathology of this type in all regions of the spine. Even arterio-venous malformations are more often than not MRI-detectable, though this is one situation where myelography still has a part to play. Occasionally also in disc disease, the surgeon will request a radiculogram after MRI to confirm underfilling of the implicated roots which cannot be seen on MRI.

In patients with clinically definite MS, about 75% will show one or more intrinsic cord lesions,[13] usually smaller than one cm in length, and as reflected in clinical and pathological studies, mostly in the cervical cord. An acute spinal cord syndrome may be associated with a lesion which is several segments in length or with multiple lesions throughout the cervical cord, and cord swelling may be apparent, occasionally making differentiation from tumor difficult. In these circumstances, the demonstration of associated brain lesions is helpful. In clinically partial syndromes, it is often surprising that the extent of disability is not much greater when one sees the extent of cord involvement. New spinal cord lesions appear in a ratio of about one in ten in comparison to cerebral lesions, but they are more likely to be symptomatic, presumably because of the lack of functionally redundant tissue in the cord.

The demonstration of spinal lesions may also be of value in making the diagnosis, particularly in older patients, in whom the brain appearances may be age-related or non-specific. This situation highlights the limitation of MRI in more elderly patients, particularly those over 55 in whom deep white matter "lesions" are commonly found which are probably vascular in origin and of no pathological significance. In these people, there is a case for seeking other evidence of the nature of the disease and of dissemination by means of evoked potentials and lumbar puncture.

The optic nerve is another part of the CNS amenable to study by MRI. Using appropriate imaging techniques, mainly aimed at suppressing the signal from orbital fat, the nerve can be clearly visualized and, to some extent, its MRI characteristics quantified. In acute optic neuritis, over 80% of affected nerves will show high signal on conventional images. With the use of special receiver coils placed over the eyes, this figure is now nearer 100%, making the technique as sensitive as VEP, but with the added advantage that the lesion can be seen and measured. The acute lesion consistently shows Gd enhancement,[14] which usually lasts for the same length of time as elsewhere in the CNS, and the appearance of the lesion evolves over months in a way consistent with the known pathophysiology as described in section 5.3 above.

As with imaging of the spinal cord, however, the main value of MRI of the orbits is for excluding other lesions which may mimic optic neuritis or cause a progressive optic neuropathy. For example, a commoner syndrome in the more elderly patient in whom the diagnosis of optic neuritis is being considered is anterior ischemic optic neuropathy.

MRI can distinguish the two conditions with useful precision on the basis that in the ischemic neuropathy, the lesion is at the nerve head, so imaging of the nerve will be normal at a time when optic neuritis consistently causes signal change. Other pathological processes which enter into the differential diagnosis of optic neuritis will be discussed in Chapter 6.

MULTIPLE SCLEROSIS

It is no exaggeration to say that MRI has, in the last 15 years revolutionized our thinking in MS, and in has a number of roles in addition to those already mentioned, which are discussed later in this book. Among the more important are prognostication, assessing specific clinical deficits and disabilities and monitoring of the efficacy of new treatments in therapeutic trials.

5.7 How does MRI help in Monitoring MS?

This question is of some importance for the assessment of new treatments aimed at modifying the natural history of the disease. It is beyond the scope of this book to describe the techniques in detail, but worthy of mention that several new methods of measuring disease activity, particularly in combination, are proving more sensitive and specific for the evaluation of the efficacy of new treatments at the pathological level.

In addition to established techniques such as T_1-enhanced images and T_2 lesion load, among the most promising are:

- MTR ratios whereby loss of tissue may be measured

- MR Spectroscopy, which measures metabolic components of tissue, and therefore their derangement, for example with established axonal loss and irrecoverable disability

- Brain parenchymal fraction (BPF), which monitors the overall loss of brain tissue

Although unrelated to MRI, it is also appropriate to note at this point, that other means of monitoring disease activity also show promise, including the detection and measurement of myelin basic protein-like material (MBPLM) in urine, and better methods of clinical assessment.

CHAPTER 6

THE CLINICAL PATTERNS OF MS

6.1 How do we classify patients with Multiple Sclerosis?

At one time MS was MS. Some patients deteriorated faster than others sometimes episodically and sometimes steadily; some seemed not to deteriorate at all. Although most did relapse and remit, a few patients did not. It has always been apparent that the majority of patients who developed the disease in early adult life showed a relapsing and remitting clinical course, RRMS, which varies greatly in severity from individual to individual. Following a relapsing-remitting onset a proportion of patients were known to enter a secondary phase of steady progression with or without superimposed relapses, or SPMS. Furthermore, for want of a better name, and because of the presence of oligoclonal bands in some patients, a separate category of MS was recognized in which clinical course was steadily progressive and without relapses from onset. This category was initially classified together with the secondary progressive form of the disease as chronic progressive MS, but in the past decade has been more clearly delineated on good scientific grounds as a separate category known as primary progressive MS (PPMS).[15]

The final categories which deserve separate consideration from the other groups are benign and malignant (Marburg's disease) MS. The classification currently most popular is therefore predominantly based on clinical observations of the natural history of the disease, and does not attempt to imply or infer etiological or even pathological mechanisms. It is to be hoped, however, that future work will allow a reclassification based on more fundamental, perhaps immunopathological properties of the disease or (more likely) diseases with relevance to specific treatments or prognosis or both.

From Table 6.1 it can be seen that the majority of patients will present with an attack or relapse of the disease. At this stage the patient has an isolated clinical syndrome of the type seen in MS but cannot, of course be diagnosed after a single attack.

MULTIPLE SCLEROSIS

Category of MS	(% of total)	Definition
1 BENIGN	(10-20%)	No significant disability due to MS 10 years after onset (EDSS* three or less)
2 RRMS	(45%)	Clearly defined relapses (with or without remissions) from onset. Any fixed disability entirely due to incomplete recovery from relapses. No evidence of progression between relapses
3 SPMS	(40%)	Initially relapsing-remitting then develops into steadily progressive course with or without superimposed relapses, minor remissions and plateaus
4 PPMS	(5-10%)	Disease progressive from onset with minor plateaus and temporary improvements allowed, but no clear relapses

(Some authors include a further category of chronic-relapsing MS, defined as relapses superimposed upon an apparently primary progressive course, but this is of dubious validity)

Table 6.1   Types of MS based of natural history

* Kurtzke's Expanded Disability Status Scale

6.2 Is disability inevitable?

In benign MS, the patient accumulates no significant disability ten years after onset, and so is a retrospective diagnosis (or prognosis if you guess the patient has it before ten years have elapsed). There are often clear indications within the first couple of years that the disease will follow a benign course. In general, such patients have infrequent relapses, not necessarily mild, but with a tendency to affect mainly sensory (including optic nerve) functions. Although only about 10-20% fall strictly into the benign category with no disability after ten years, as many as a third of patients overall have no or minor problems after this disease duration. Predicting benign disease is not a precise science in the early stages. However, when compared to the other MS categories in whom only 12% are symptom-free within a month of the first attack (pre-diagnosis), 37% of those who go on to develop benign disease reach this desirable state.[16] If the MRI of the brain shows minimal or no changes early in the disease, then a benign outcome is more likely.

It is also held that involvement of only one neurological system in the initial attack is a strong predictor of a benign course,[17] a conclusion about which there must be some reservations given the rather higher frequency of monosymptomatic attacks at onset than of benign MS.[18] Furthermore, even ten years after onset the diagnosis of benign disease can be misleading. One unusual clinical course involved a man who had three sensory relapses with full recovery in his 20s, correctly diagnosed as clinically definite MS, only to develop, in his late 40s, a series of devastating motor attacks which left him severely and permanently disabled. He is the exception rather than the rule, but illustrates that this heinous disease can always mislead us, and we might expect any eventuality.

6.3 What is the worst that can happen?

At the opposite end of the spectrum is the form of RRMS known as malignant MS or Marburg's disease, and is, unfortunately, likely to strike younger patients. This variant of MS is a monophasic, acute or subacute, severe demyelinating condition with a poor, often fatal outcome. Some patients deteriorate rapidly from onset, never remit and die within weeks or a few months. Others may suffer a more subacute, but no less unremitting illness, leading within several months to death or severe fixed disability. The diagnosis may not be straightforward as the onset may be rapid, so that by the time the patient reaches hospital they are in coma and the differential diagnosis is wide.

Further investigation can usually confirm the inflammatory nature of the illness, but differentiation from severe acute disseminated encephalomyelitis, aggressive lymphoma or certain infections may not be possible prior to death. Needless to say, the response to treatment is not gratifying. MRI reflects the very aggressive nature of the disease, showing widespread cerebral white matter involvement which may, in the worst cases, have the appearance of, and behave like multiple mass lesions, and even lead to a cerebral herniation syndrome refractory to treatment.

A similar fulminant episode in the illness may arise in patients who have been in a progressive phase for years,an observation strongly supportive of the argument that the Marburg variant is a true form of MS. Pathologically also, the findings are consistent with severe, acute MS: within the lesions demyelination is extensive and loss of axons may be conspicuous. The associated inflammatory changes and vasogenic edema, likewise, are extreme, unless modified by steroid and other therapy prior to death. Fortunately, Marburg's disease is very uncommon. Physicians with an interest may expect to come across no more than two or three such patients in any five year period.

6.4 But What Usually Happens?

Including those with benign MS, 90% or more of patients show a relapsing-remitting course from onset.[16] A typical relapse is characterized by the appearance of new or recrudescence of old symptoms for a period greater than 24 hours. In practice, relapses are usually easily recognized by the patient and last several weeks. In fact, despite the above definition, it would be suspicious if symptoms only lasted 24 hours that there was some other cause for the patient's complaint. Having an inflammatory basis, relapses generally progress over a few days or weeks before stabilizing for a further few weeks and then recovery follows. A mild relapse may recovery fully within a week, a more severe one may not recover at all.

Interestingly, patients commonly experience a minor recurrence of old symptoms at the time of an anatomically distinct relapse. For example, an attack referable to the cervical cord may be accompanied by mild blurring of vision in an eye previously affected by optic neuritis. The explanation is unclear, but perhaps this phenomenon reflect a more generalized process within the CNS mediated by blood-borne factors. Patients who notice this type of symptom can be reassured that it will certainly clear regardless of what happens to the main relapse.

It is an interesting clinical observation that in any one patient, the nature of relapses tends to be stereotyped. For example, it would be surprising, if, having jogged along quite nicely for years with relatively mild sensory attacks, a patient suddenly threw of a severe paraplegia or ataxic episode. Conversely, a series of malicious motor attacks is unlikely to give way to episodes of tingling limbs.

Exceptions to this rule tend to stick in the mind: a different patient to the one described under "Benign" MS above (SD) had three attacks of optic neuritis and one of sensory impairment between the ages of 21 and 25. A clinically definite diagnosis of MS was made. He then experienced no new symptoms for 14 years and clearly had benign disease. At the age of 39, however, he developed, overnight, a paraplegia which only recovered following steroid therapy to the point where he could walk with a stick. Five months later, it recurred with little recovery and he is now permanently wheelchair-bound and has significant bladder dysfunction. Further investigation confirmed the cause to be MS. It seemed that he had developed the disease twice in one lifetime!

Some types of attack have a better prognosis than others for satisfactory recovery: for example, optic neuritis and most other purely sensory attacks will do well, as, symptomatically, will attacks producing true vertigo or double vision; ataxia and bladder disturbances on the other hand tend to cause some degree of residual or recurring deficit and often disability. Generally, also, good recovery from attacks tends to augur better for the future. Prognostication in MS will be considered in more detail in Chapter 8.

Always within the limitations of the well-known heterogeneity of the disease between individuals, the general trend is for relapses in the earlier years to recover more satisfactorily. At this stage the annual relapse frequency averages around 2-2.5. Thereafter, the frequency of relapses tends to fall gradually over the years, but recovery from them tends to be less complete, and it is at this stage that the patient begins to accumulate fixed disability. In general, most MS attacks will be mild.

In the pivotal trial of interferon ß-1b (see Chapter 12), mild attacks appeared at a rate of 0.54/year, whereas moderate and severe attacks occurred less frequently at 0.45/year. Factors predictive of recovery include rapidity of onset: the more rapid the better the recovery: sensory attacks tend to leave less residual disability: attacks occurring on a background of SPMS tend to recover less well in response to steroids, and satisfactory recovery becomes less likely to occur more than a month into the attack.

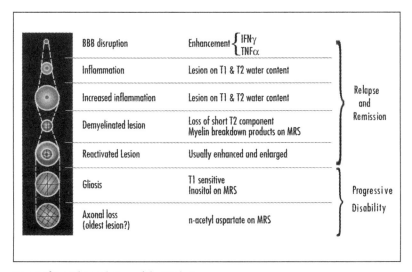

Figure 6.1a: The evolution of the MS lesion

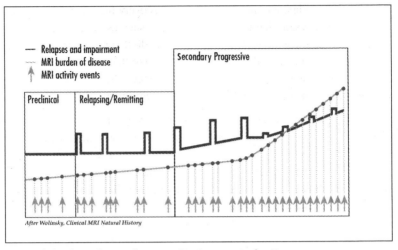

Figure 6.1b: The evolution of RRMS to SPMS in a typical patient

6.5 What is meant by the progressive phase?

Although it is not uncommon for MS sufferers to become significantly disabled in the long-term purely through incomplete recovery of their relapses, it is the supervention of SPMS which causes most concern among doctors experienced in looking after these people. If about one third of all RRMS follows a benign or only mildly disabling clinical course, then the majority of the rest, about 40% at six years and 50-60% more than ten years after onset will enter a secondarily progressive phase; this figure rises further with an even longer disease duration.

SPMS is defined as progression of clinical disability (with or without relapses and minor fluctuation) after a relapsing-remitting onset. Of all the prognostic indicators of outcome in RRMS, the subsequent development of SPMS carries the most certain promise of more severe disability. It is often difficult to define the point at which an individual patient converts from RR to SPMS. Only in retrospect can the patient say that for a certain length of time, in the absence of relapses, they would have got worst anyway. It usually takes at least six months of progression before the situation becomes clear.

The physician must take care here: to conclude that the patient has developed SPMS is to condemn them to certain worsening disability. It is important to wait long enough to be sure that progression is indeed due to a worsening baseline and not to incomplete recovery from attacks or a perceived progression due to some other cause such as depression or the appearance of fatigue or some confounding medical condition. Once diagnosed with certainty, the physician must make the time to discuss the implications of the diagnosis with the patient since it is, in effect, a new disease state. This aspect of management is often forgotten.

The majority of patients entering the secondary progressive phase of the illness will develop substantial disability and lose physical independence within a further ten years. At this stage there will almost invariable be involvement of motor pathways causing walking difficulties, some disturbance of bladder and sexual function, and possibly pain, speech disorders and visual problems as described later in this Chapter.

6.6 What is primary progressive MS?

PPMS is defined as the form of MS characterized by progressive disability from onset, without relapses and remissions. Thus, although the clinical course may show minor fluctuations from time to time, the unfortunate sufferer experiences a steadily worsening level of disability with little hope of respite. This form of the disease is relatively uncommon, representing no more than 5-10% of the MS population, but tends to occur in the older age group (typical onset 5th and 6th decades) and, for a given duration of disease, cause greater levels of disability. Clearly, in the absence of relapses and remissions, the diagnostic emphasis must, more than ever, focus on the exclusion of other types of pathology that might present with progressive symptoms and signs.

The site of neurological involvement is most commonly the cervical cord resulting in a progressive spastic paraparesis, though other manifestations might include a progressive brainstem syndrome, or even less commonly, monocular visual failure or progressive cerebellar ataxia. In these circumstances, MRI is particularly useful in excluding commoner causes of these syndromes such as spondylotic myelopathy, syringomyelia, space-occupying lesions and primary neurodegenerative disease. This circumstance also may justify a lumbar puncture to confirm, as far as possible, the immune and inflammatory nature of the condition, since the usual Poser criteria cannot be applied to this type of MS.

It is unexplained why the brain MRI in patients with PPMS is likely to demonstrate far less lesion load for a given disease duration than either

MULTIPLE SCLEROSIS

RRMS or SPMS. More specialist techniques, however, may be helpful, including cross-sectional imaging of the cervical cord, where there is clear evidence for a correlation between cord atrophy and prognosis for disability in these patients. As mentioned above, PPMS generally carries a poor prognosis for disability and no formal treatment trials have shown benefit, though this is partly because there are fewer patients to study, and to profit from!. There are finally, however, trials underway looking at the clinical tolerability and efficacy of Interferon ß-1a in PPMS. At present, in most parts of the world, physicians can either confine themselves to offering appropriate symptomatic management or considering the use of azathioprine, as the only drug currently available which might help some patients with more aggressive disease despite the lack of objective data to support its use.

CHAPTER 7

THE CLINICAL MANIFESTATIONS OF MS

7.1 How does MS usually start?

So-called "sites of predilection" of the demyelinating process dictate the commonest types of relapse at onset. The optic nerves, cervical cord and brainstem including cerebellar peduncles seem, for reasons so far unclear to bear the brunt of this process, though it may be no coincidence that these are all sites with little if any non-eloquent neural elements, and so symptoms are almost inevitable with even small plaques in these regions.

Commonly, the first attack is of optic neuritis. The severity will vary from virtually asymptomatic to complete blindness with little recovery. The typical attack begins with pain behind the affected eye which worsens over a day or two, may be severe and is most prominent on eye movement. At about the same time or shortly after, the patient develops a visual disturbance usually affecting the center of vision most prominently, and worsens over days until useful acuity is lost. Often color appreciation is differentially affected at onset, and it is remarkable how many affected individuals cannot lateralize or may not even notice quite marked visual loss, and only complain of the pain. Acuity is affected without pain in 58% of cases. The condition may worsen for a few hours (30%), days (50%), or weeks and then stabilize. As the days pass the pain tends to improve, and it

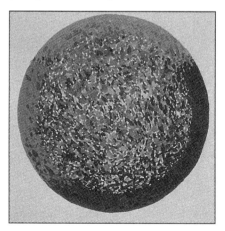

Figure 7.1: A depiction of optic neuritis as seen by the artist Peter McCarrol as he attempted to obey the instruction of his neurologist to "look at my voice"

is usual for the worst of the discomfort to be gone within a week to ten days of onset. Visual recovery is more gradual, often continuing for six weeks or even longer, though if there has been no useful visual recovery after four weeks, then the ultimate prognosis is less clear. Overall, more than 90% of patients recover acuity to 6/9 (20/30).

Phosphenes (visual flashes with eye movement) may be noticed by some patients, and other symptoms after the recovery phase include Uhthoff's phenomenon whereby acuity in a previously affected eye worsens transiently with exercise or other causes of raised body temperature such as a hot bath or shower. The Pulfrich effect which can be prominent and disconcerting in some, and consists of an illusion of curved motion of an object actually moving in a straight line. For example, a car approaching on the other side of the road can appear, somewhat alarmingly, to be driving purposefully across the center of the road towards the unfortunate sufferer. Clinically, this effect can be demonstrated by swinging a pendulum (usually a tendon hammer) from side to side in front of the patient who will observe an elliptical component to the linear swing. This effect is explained by the mismatch of conduction speeds from the two eyes upsetting the normally balanced binocular judgement of velocity.

Clinical findings during the acute attack may be unremarkable. It has been said of optic neuritis that "the patient sees nothing and the physician sees nothing". If the inflammation is in the retrobulbar portion of the nerve, then the optic disc will be swollen, and possibly associated with exudates and perivenular cuffing out on the fundus, but hemorrhage is only occasionally apparent (no more than 5% of cases). The signs are otherwise those of an optic neuropathy, with a relative afferent pupillary defect (when a bright light is swung from eye to eye each second) and impaired acuity, particularly central. Color perception, however, may be selectively impaired, with acuity relatively spared. There may also be tenderness on globe pressure, but proptosis is uncommonly if ever seen, even in severe attacks. Very occasionally optic neuritis runs a slowly progressive course resulting in gradual visual failure over months or years in the affected eye.

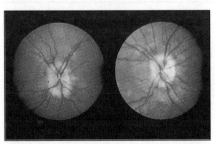

Figure 7.2: Optic disc swelling (arrowed) in actute retrobulbar neuritis

After the acute stage, the residual signs correlate with the degree of recovery. A mild attack will leave, at best, subtle signs in the affected eye, such as sluggish reading of the Ishihara color plates; a moderate attack may also produce a degree of optic atrophy, a persistent afferent pupillary defect and a loss of color appreciation as well as a mild drop in acuity. A severe attack (perhaps 5% of cases) may be followed by little or no useful recovery. The prognosis may not be apparent from the clinical features of the attack, but does correlate with the MRI appearances of physically long lesions in the optic nerve and also with the location of the lesion in the bony optic canal, presumably because the nerve is more severely compressed at this site.

For this reason, the management of optic neuritis may include a course of steroids, which are best reserved for those patients with a severe drop in acuity or severe pain, and for those with impaired vision in the fellow eye because of the greater risk of visual disability if recovery is not complete. Otherwise, evidence that steroids effect ultimate visual prognosis is lacking. If MRI of the optic nerves is undertaken, as it might be if the diagnosis is in doubt, and the lesion is long or in the optic canal, then a course of steroids is indicated.

In the rare instances of simultaneous bilateral optic neuritis associated with MS, steroids are also usually prescribed. In most cases of optic neuritis, however, the use of steroids remains controversial. One of the largest trial to date was undertaken by Beck and colleagues.[16] They randomized 457 patients to receive either oral prednisone (1 mg/kg body weight per day for 14 days), intravenous methylprednisolone (1 gm daily for three days) followed by oral prednisone (1 mg/kg per day for 11 days) or oral placebo for 14 days. Visual function was assessed over a six month period. Recovery was fastest in the group receiving intravenous methylprednisolone. This was particularly true for the reversal of visual field defects, but other functions, including contrast sensitivity, color vision and acuity also benefited. By six months, however, the efficacy of steriods was much diminished, and there were no significant differences between the oral prednisone

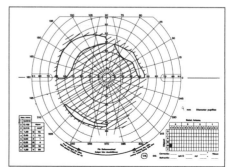

Figure 7.3: Goldmann Fields showing typical central scotoma of optic neuritis

MULTIPLE SCLEROSIS

Clinical feature	At presentation	At any time
Visual	49	100
Diplopia	12	31
Weakness	43	89
Sensory	41	87
Ataxia	23	82
Sphincter/sexual	10	63
Cognitive	4	39

Table 7.1   Prevalence of clinical features at onset and during course of MS

and placebo group. The bottom line seems to be that, as with other types of demyelinating episodes, steroids hasten recovery from optic neuritis, but make only a marginal, if any difference to the eventual outcome.

Other aims of management include a full explanation of the condition and its generally excellent prognosis; the use of analgesics, as strong as required, and the exclusion of other possible diagnoses as appropriate, though some form of imaging will be required in patients with no relevant past history of neurological episodes.

7.2 What are the commonest manifestations?

Here, some of the more important disabling clinical manifestations of MS will be discussed in no particular order. The interested reader should consult a specialist text for a more comprehensive description of all the features of the disease since such a description is beyond the scope of this book.

The question of what is or is not a typical manifestation of MS is of the utmost importance. A familiarity with the typical clinical deficits of demyelination enables the recognition of atypical or frankly unacceptable features for of the disease. In MS, hemiplegia at or soon after onset, for example, is very uncommon, as are central visual defects such as a homonymous hemianopia. These features are, of course, more likely to be the result of vascular disease, but may be acceptable for MS provided the commoner causes have been excluded. It used to be said that everyone with MS will experience some problem with their vision or sensation or sphincter function at some time, and this aphorism is worthy of consideration even today. Such symptoms may fluctuate markedly, particularly in the first few years after onset of the disease.

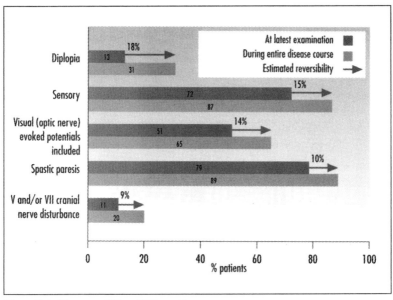

Figure 7.4: The reversibility of MS symptoms

7.2.1 Sensory symptoms

Sensory symptoms are very common early in the course of the disease, probably more so than suggested by the data given in Table 7.1. It is the sensory symptoms and signs that cause the most difficulty when it comes to assessing diagnostic value. Patients often confuse feeling with strength and so declare a numb or clumsy hand to be "weak", even though muscular strength is normal. The the most reliable symptoms of sensory involvement are definite numbness, pins and needles, tightness around a limb (implying posterior column involvement) and a sensation of water spilling down a limb (probably spinothalamic). Other relatively common, though often vague 'sensory' symptoms, including 'hot', 'cold', and 'shuddering' and 'juddering' are not necessarily indicative of damage to sensory pathways; indeed their origin usually remains obscure. Such symptoms may, however, be distressing to patients and, which reassurance is appropriate; they should not be trivialized.

M ULTIPLE SCLEROSIS

When MS is established, it is very unusual for there to be no sensory problems, though in general they are not particularly disabling. Exceptions include severe deafferentation where joint position appreciation is lost and the hand in particular will be numb and clumsy and lack the discrete fine movement need for fine manipulation (Oppenheimer hand). Most patients quickly learn to compensate for sensory disturbances or to ignore persistent tingles so that disability is mild.

More disturbing to the patient are painful sensory symptoms. Patients commonly experience such symptoms when there is damage from the disease to the posterior columns in the cervical spinal cord, which produces a feeling of a "tight band" or constriction around the limbs or more often trunk, sometimes even making breathing difficult. Other examples include painful limb dysesthesia and deep boring pains due to the sensory myelopathic process. Unlike diseases of the peripheral nervous system, these patients usually have relatively minor sensory signs clinically.

7.2.2 Motor Symptoms

Motor symptoms are common in MS, and generally more disabling than sensory problems (Table 7.1). Problems with movement may result from increased muscle tone, weakness, clumsiness and tremor and other abnormal involuntary movements. As with all aspects of the clinical history, however, it is important, when listening to the patient, to ascertain exactly what is being described. Patients often confuse motor and sensory symptoms: they may, for example, say that a limb is 'numb' when it is weak, but much more commonly will say a limb is 'weak' when, actually it is affected by a sensory disturbance. Nevertheless, true motor features are the most common cause of physical disability in patients with MS.

White matter disease in general tends to produce considerable spasticity that may, or may not, be accompanied by weakness. Following an acute attack of MS, weakness may recover, but leave the limb spastic. With the clear exception of cerebellar ataxia, it is spasticity which causes the greatest difficulty with motor function in MS. It may be accompanied by spasms, often painful and nocturnal, and in response to a stimulus. These spasms usually interfere with function, and in more disabled people, make handling be the carer very difficult, the management of spasticity and spasms will be discussed later. It is important to remember, however, that suppression of spasticity by muscle relaxants may be counterproductive to function. A patient may walk with difficulty, but remain ambulatory because of the support provided by leg spasticity. If that stiffness is relieved by drug therapy, the weakened leg(s) may no longer be able to carry the body weight, and an ambulatory individual would require a wheelchair. It is, therefore, of the utmost importance continually to review the situation in such patients, preferably with the help of the physiotherapists, as described in Chapter 9.

Spasticity in the arms is usually of less functional importance than in the legs, but when there is bilateral damage to the corticospinal pathways above the medulla, the patient will develop a pseudobulbar palsy. This disorder, like other forms of spasticity is characterized by slowness, stiffness and hyperreflexia of the affected muscles. Speech becomes slow and labored, and its sound has been likened, not inappropriately to "eating a hot potato". Swallowing may be affected, and the brisk gag reflex causes regurgitation of food through the nose. Fortunately, unlike its dreaded lower motor neuron equivalent, the bulbar palsy, a pseudobulbar palsy rarely causes aspiration of food, by virtue of the briskness of the bulbar reflexes. When severe and progressive, however, it will eventually render the sufferer anarthric and unable to swallow.

Pure weakness without spasticity is uncommon in MS but may occur. Occasionally, also, one may see lower motor neuron signs despite this disease being confined to the CNS. In the cervical spinal cord, for example, an MS lesion may involve the anterior horn cell projections at one or more levels resulting in focal wasting, weakness and loss of the appropriate deep tendon reflexes, mimicking and difficult to differentiate clinically from degenerative disease or a disc lesion. MS tends to affect the small hand muscles more than these other conditions.

Needless to say, someone suffering from MS is in no way protected against other, potentially treatable diseases, and it is important to bear this point in mind, and investigating as appropriate with, for example, MRI, given the possibility of successful intervention. Unfortunately, this clinical scenario is usually attributable to severe involvement of the cervical cord by demyelination, and accompanied by substantial and progressive arm disability.

In general, the most disabling manifestation of motor system dysfunction is cerebellar involvement. It is well established that when the cerebellar pathways are affected early in the disease, the prognosis for both disability and early death is poor. Most commonly cerebellar symptoms involve the limbs, walking balance and speech. These features may arise as part of an acute attack, often with other brainstem features, or more ominously, emerge gradually in the course of SPMS.

One of the most distressing symptoms of this type is an intention tremor. In the context of good muscle power and intact sensation the affected individual is quite unable to carry out any useful movement because the limb oscillates from side to side with ever greater amplitude as the target is approached. in extreme cases this can even cause injury.

As the patient attempts to pick up an object, the arm swings violently in an arc striking anything in the way be it a heavy or sharp object or even the patient's own face. Such extreme examples are mercifully uncommon, but even relatively mild cerebellar involvement may make carrying a cup of hot liquid hazardous. When it affects the midline structures this type of ataxia causes a characteristic broad-based gait with unpredictable lurching from side to side as if drunk. These patients in general, have difficulty with simple and more complex motor tasks such as dressing, and are dependent on carers despite other functions being spared.

Apart from tremor, abnormal involuntary movements are uncommon in MS but do occur, mainly secondary to involvement by the disease of the basal ganglia. Such movements include chorea and myoclonic jerks. A benign form is myokymia: this muscular twitch is almost universal from time to time in normal individuals, consisting of an irritating twitch usually repetitive and affecting an eyelid. In MS, it may be more persistent and visible, and has led patients to seek advice about how it might be suppressed, for example using botulinum toxin. Epilepsy is also more common in patients with MS than in the general population; approximately 2-5% of sufferers will experience more than one seizure as opposed to a prevalence of epilepsy in people without MS of 0.5%.

7.2.3 Eye movement disorders

Up to three-quarters of patients with MS will demonstrate one type of eye movement disorder or another during the course of their disease, and examination of a patient with suspected or established MS cannot be complete without a careful assessment of ocular motility.[19] The most common problems overall, are those associated with cerebellar involvement. Dysmetria is the commonest and may be accompanied by nystagmus of various types.

The most characteristic eye movement abnormality in MS, however, is the internuclear ophthalmoplegia (INO), which is, simply defined, a slowing of adduction. In other words as the patient looks quickly to one side, the adducting eye lags behind its abducting fellow. Most INOs are associated with additional clinical features including some impairment of vertical, particularly upward gaze, a few beats of large amplitude (ataxic) nystagmus in the abducting eye. In some more severe examples, adduction is both slow and incomplete, the affected eye coming to rest some way short of full medical gaze. Regardless of these other features, however, when the clinician can demonstrate a relative slowing of adduction, the "diagnosis" of an INO is confirmed.

As mentioned above, involvement of vertical gaze is almost universal with an INO, because the medial longitudinal fasciculus (MLF), being the site of the lesion causing a unilateral INO, carries fibers important for vertical gaze to the rostral interstitial nucleus of the medial longitudinal fasciculus. More than 50% of INOs are bilateral, though one side may be subtle. Note that a left sided INO will be seen by asking the patient to look to the right and vice versa. An important clinical point here is that to see the slowed adduction it is necessary to look at the bridge of the patient's nose as they look quickly from side to side, between two targets held at 30 degrees at either side of the midline; it is likely that, unless it is severe, an INO will be missed if the examination is confined to the testing of slow phase (smooth pursuit), eye movement only.

It is surprisingly uncommon for patients to be symptomatic from an INO, but when they are, the most characteristic description is of their brain not keeping up with their eye, or feeling momentarily disorientated one looking to the affected side. Double vision is distinctly rare even with incomplete adduction.

Other common eye movement problems associated with MS include pendular nystagmus and ocular flutter. In the former, the eyes oscillate about a point with equal speed in all directions, much as a pendulum will when perturbed. This may occur in any plane, and may be linear or even circular. Unfortunately there is often associated oscillopsia, the symptom of movement of what is seen corresponding to the movement of the eyes, which can be very disabling to vision. This symptom may, however, respond to treatment with either baclofen or gabapentin.

Visual symptoms associated with abnormal involuntary eye movements are mercifully uncommon. Ocular flutter is a useful sign of brainstem involvement in which the eye suddenly and conjugately flick in the horizontal plane and back again without a pause. If these movements also involve the vertical plane, they are called opsoclonus: the latter however, is less common in MS and is more an indication of either viral or paraneoplastic brainstem disease.

7.2.4 Bladder, bowel and sexual problems

Like sensory and visual syndromes, problems with bladder function are both characteristic of and very common in MS (see Figure 7.5).[20] Broadly speaking, they are of two types: bladder hyperreflexia and detruso-sphincter dyssernygia (DSD).

The first describes the typical disorder of bladder function where the patient experiences urgency, frequency, nocturnal disturbances and urge incontinence. These problems arise because the bladder, analogous to spasticity and hyperreflexia elsewhere, and usually associated with them, cannot relax sufficiently to allow normal filling. As the bladder fills, it starts to contract at much smaller

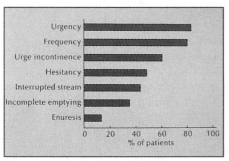

Figure 7.5: The prevalence of bladder disturbances in MS

volumes than normal due to hyperreflexia. The sufferer notices that the urge to pass urine comes too frequently, and that they are unable to delay micturition due to urgency, which will result in incontinence if they cannot void quickly. In the more severe cases, there is almost no warning, and incontinence is inevitable. This affliction leads to considerable handicap. Trips out have to be planned around toilets. They cannot visit public places unless they know there is relief nearby, and sleep is frequently disturbed by the need to get out of bed to pass urine. Urodynamics demonstrate the typical changes of a poorly compliant bladder with the rapid build-up of intravesical pressure with relatively small volumes and associated contractions of the detrusor appear at abnormal low volumes. Fortunately, this type of bladder disturbance is amenable to treatment with bladder relaxants as described later.

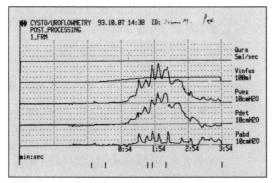

Figure 7.6: The evolution of the MS lesion

It is important to remember that bladder spasticity of this type is unusual without similar spasticity in the legs: indeed in the absence of the latter, the former rarely occurs in spinal disease of any type.

The second characteristic type of bladder problem in MS is detrusor-sphincter dyssernygia. In this disorder, bladder hyperreflexia is associated with an inability to relax the external voluntary sphincter during micturition. The symptoms which result are predictable and consist of a delay or inability to initiate voiding, poor stream, repetitive micturition, frequency, urgency and an impression (usually correct) of incomplete bladder emptying. Thus, in addition to the inconvenience of hyperreflexia is added the frustration and discomfort of poor bladder emptying. As a result, there is often significant retention of urine and recurrent urinary tract infection, which, ultimately, may lead to serious renal complications. These patients again are often treated successfully, usually with a combination of bladder relaxants and intermittent self-catheterization (ISC), though other, more specialist input may be required.

Problems with bowel function are usually confined to constipation and should respond to normal measures. It is worth bearing in mind, however, that in MS bladder and bowel function are interrelated, and problems with one may exacerbate or even cause problems with the other, and also that many drugs used to treat the symptoms of MS may lead to constipation.

A typical sequence of events is where, as a direct result of immobility, a patient becomes constipated, and as a result of that develops worsening frequency and urgency of micturition. Correct management depends on identifying the sequence of events leading to the overall condition, not treating any one manifestation in isolation.

Disorders of sexual function are also common in MS, and the first step in their management is their identification. Patients may be naturally reluctant to mention these difficulties, so direct inquiries must be made, and a sympathetic but professional approach crucial. Anorgasmia in either men or women may well have a psychological rather than physical basis: feelings of loss of self-esteem, depression, chronic pain, and drug therapies may all contribute and are potentially correctable. Neurogenic anorgasmia is less common but untreatable. Lack of libido and erectile failure in men are more amenable to treatment by physical and pharmacological measures described in Chapter 9. The prevalence of erectile difficulties in men with MS is about 60%.

Acute Pain

    Painful tonic spasms
    Trigeminal neuralgia
    Painful Lhermitte's symptom
    Paroxysmal root and limb pain

Subacute Pain

    Pain associated with relapses eg. painful optic neuritis
    Muscular pains
    Band-like dysesthesia
    Sciatica

Chronic Pain

    Low back and other spinal pain
    Myelopathic pain (especially legs and lower trunk, but also hands and arms)
    Chronic daily headache

Other Pain

    Bladder-derived pain including painful spasms

Table 7.2   Some of the commoner pain syndromes associated with MS

The apparent increase in this figure since the first surveys of the 1920s is likely to indicate a lessening of the reluctance to mention this problem in the first place when talking to the physician or other professional. These symptoms generally follow those of bladder dysfunction, probably because erections can be produced by both sympathetic and parasympathetic pathways. In either case spinal disease is most likely to cause the disturbance.

There is little in the way of hard data concerning the physiology of ejaculation, though it is known that there is a center subserving this function at the T12-L1 level. It is most likely that MS interferes with orgasm and ejaculation in both men and women by a combination of physical and psychological factors. The former include impairment of the afferent sensory pathways from the genitalia, and the efferents from cerebral centers to do with eroticism. There is little correlation between sexual difficulties of these types and physical disability in more mildly affected individuals, but a stronger one with psychological problems and chronic pain, drug and alcohol intake and marital problems.

7.2.5 Pain syndromes in MS

About 30-65% of MS sufferers experience significant pain due to their disease (Table 7.1).[21] There are a variety of pain syndromes more common in people with MS than the general population, though of course, MS is no protection against any type of pain. Among the various types of pain in MS, the most characteristic are trigeminal neuralgia (TGN), myelopathic pain and spinal and paraspinal pain, particularly in the lower back.

TGN is 4000 times more common in MS than in aged matched unaffected individuals. Neuralgia is an over used term which identifies a very specific type of pain. It is brief, shock-like, lancinating, often excruciating and certainly cannot be ignored. It may be repetitive and knife-like. Individual neuralgic pains are never long lived, though a bout of them may be sufficiently persistent to lead to suicidal ideation in the sufferer. To add insult to injury, whereas idiopathic TGN of the elderly is unilateral, a significant proportion of MS patients experience it bilaterally at different times. TGN is one of the so-called paroxysmal manifestations of MS; others will be described later.

For reasons not clearly understood, the pain is most common in the lower two divisions of the trigeminal nerve, and rare in the ophthalmic; the opposite applies to trigeminal shingles. Note that neuralgias in MS and in general may affect virtual any individual nerve, though some are more common than others. In addition to the trigeminal, the occipital and glossopharyngeal are particularly vulnerable among the nerves of the head and neck.

The second type of pain characteristic of MS is myelopathic pain. This syndrome may be even more distressing than TGN because of its persistent nature. As a result of damage to the spinal cord sensory pathways, a variety of different types of pain may be felt in the trunk and legs. With involvement of the posterior columns (joint position and vibration by tradition), the patient experiences a very characteristic tightness around the affected part. In the legs, for example, the may describe a sensation as in someone had wound a tight bandage around the knee or ankle (usually a joint) or the leg was encased.

On the body, it is usually a sensation of chest tightness, sometimes to the point of making it difficult for the sufferer to breathe. This type of sensation, fortunately, is not usually persistent, tending to resolve with the acute relapse: persistence of this typical symptom should raise suspicion of an alternative cause, such as compressive myelopathy. More commonly, myelopathic pain is a chronic syndrome in relation to partial injury to the spinal pain pathways. This type of pain, usually most prominent in the legs, is described as burning or boring, and refuses to improve with time.

A third pain syndrome associated with typical chronic demyelination is musculoskeletal pain. Patients with MS are more likely to suffer the everyday aches and pains of poor posture and overstressed joints than the rest of us because of difficulty maintaining proper gait and sitting position and the inevitable need to overload certain joints in order to remain mobile in the presence of significant spasticity, ataxia or focal weakness. Apart from these more common pain syndromes of MS, patients are not, of course, immune from any painful condition that may afflict us all. They are, however, less able to cope with additional physical stress of this type, and so it is crucial to enquire about pain, and take a sympathetic and constructive view to its assessment and management.

7.2.6 Fatigue

Of all the symptoms of chronic progressive or stable MS that cause disability, the most common is fatigue.[22] In general clinical practice, fatigue is an overused term: indeed it is often used quite inappropriately. By definition, fatigue implies a deterioration in performance with continuing effort, whereas the 'chronic fatigue syndrome' with which most of us are all too familiar, is usually applied to patients who are better described as 'tired all the time', or TATT for short!

The symptoms as experienced by patients with MS, however, is true fatigue. There are a number of different types in MS, and considerable variations in terms of severity, but they call all be disabling. Fatigue, as a sense of physical exhaustion with little effort, may make it impossible for the patient to achieve anything at all after lunchtime, or simply cause all activity to be associated with an excessive effort to achieve it. At its extreme, the fatigue associated with MS may be totally debilitating; in this case it represents one of the few causes of a true state of 'chronic fatigue'.

It is important when assessing this symptom to characterize it carefully so as to manage it appropriately: the patient may use the term "fatigue" generally to describe a variety of difficulties which might include depression,drowsiness due to poor night-time sleep, spasticity and stiffness due to upper motor neuron involvement, or muscular weakness. The true fatigue of MS, however, may exist with none of these, and is characteristic and difficult to treat.

7.2.7 Other paroxysmal symptoms

A number of typical clinical features of MS are of a paroxysmal type, which means that they are brief, shock-like and self-limiting, though may be expected to appear under certain circumstances or with particular provoking manouevres.[23] TGN and other neuralgias have already been mentioned as paroxysmal symptoms of MS, but others include Lhermitte's symptom (it is not a 'sign'), painful tonic spasms (PTS) and paroxysmal diplopia, dysarthria or ataxia. Lhermitte's symptom is common in MS and also in other irritative lesions involving the cervical spinal cord, and is described as a sensation, often shooting or electric, down the spine or limbs on flexing the head forward on the neck. It is thought to be due to mechanical stretching of the cord leading to ephaptic (short-circuit) transmission between partially demyelinated fibers adjacent to each other. This basis probably underlies the other paroxysmal symptoms of MS.

PTS, although fairly common in MS, are of uncertain origin. The patient experiences sudden, often very powerful and distressing spasms affecting one or many muscle groups in a limb. The leg may straighten or, less commonly flex up into the trunk, or the arm be forced against the chest. These spasms may be brief or last a few minutes if the spasm cannot be broken. Some occur spontaneously, though usually the spasm is provoked by some stimulus such as a change in position of the limb, or even a sudden noise or visual stimulus may bring on a spasm. The site of the damage in the CNS which generates these spasms has not been consistently reported, but most likely they may be caused by lesions in varied sites along the motor pathway. MRI correlations, hampered somewhat by the multifocal nature of the disease, have demonstrated a relationship between spasms and damage to the pyramidal tracts in the internal capsules and upper spinal cord, as well as in the basal ganglia.

Lhermitte's symptom may persist or even appear after the other manifestations of an attack of cervical myelitis, whether in the context of MS or not. Paroxysmal diplopia, although uncommon, can be distressing and disabling particular with respect to driving. Because of the supposed pathophysiology of these phenomena, the antiepileptic drugs have been tried, often successfully to suppress them. Carbamazepine in particular is effective and well tolerated for TGN and Lhermitte's symptom, the two most common of these symptoms.

Although uncommon in MS, epilepsy occurs more frequently in affected individuals than in the general population. It may appear as a transient phenomenon associated with a new demyelinating lesion in an eloquent part of the cerebral cortex such as the motor strip, or an a permanent complication of the disease. Both cerebral biopsy material and MRI have shown correlations between transient seizures and large, actively inflamed areas of cortical involvement, sometimes resembling tumor (pseudotumoral MS), and between permanent epilepsy and gliotic inactive demyelinated plaques.

7.2.8 Summary and atypical features

In summary, the clinical presentation of multiple sclerosis and the subsequent natural history, both with respect to the timing and nature of symptoms and signs of MS, are extremely variable and notoriously unpredictable. Any part of the CNS may be affected, but the experienced clinician will recognize that some symptoms and signs are uncommon or atypical of MS, and might raise the possibility of an alternative diagnosis in the early stages. Such symptoms and signs include hemiparesis and hemianopia. Both are very common manifestations of vascular disease, but are uncommon in the earlier stages of MS, and should ring warning bells and suggest that perhaps the patient has a vasculitis or stroke but not demyelination.

Descriptive factor	% answering yes		
	MS (n=32)	NHI (n=33)	P value
Worsened by heat	92	17	<0.001
Comes on easily	82	22	<0.001
Interferes with physical functioning	79	28	<0.01
Cases frequent problems	63	17	<0.001
Prevents sustained physical functioning	89	0	<0.001
Interferes with responsibility	67	0	<0.001

Table 7.3: Factors discriminating fatigue in MS and normal healthy individuals (NHI) *(Courtesy of Dr L B Krupp)*

7.3 What factors might trigger attacks?

The majority of relapses in MS appear for no apparent reason of within a few weeks of a non-specific, probably viral, illness. Viruses are known to trigger MS relapses, though the mechanisms by which this happens are unclear. It is known that IFN-γ increases the frequency of relapses; indeed a clinical therapeutic trial of this substance had to be stopped because of the increased relapse rate among patients on the active drug. It is also known that IFN-ß release is stimulated by viral infections, as are a number of other cytokines, which may promote the immunological changes, which lead to the development of new lesions in MS. Some vaccinations containing live, attenuated viruses have been implicated, but others like tetanus toxoid or hepatitis A immunoglobulin are probably safe.

When advising patients about vaccinations prior to travel abroad, it is a matter of balancing the potential benefits against the drawbacks. If the patient is visiting a region of high polio prevalence, for example, it is probably worth accepting the small risk of provoking a relapse to ensure protection against such a serious disease. Other trigger factors are less well identified, but many patients are persuaded that certain circumstances apply to them, such as periods of psychological distress or fatigue, though there is no good evidence in support of these as trigger in MS patients in general.

Because of the fact that most patients with MS are women of childbearing age, the relationship between disease activity and the periods of pregnancy and the puerperium is an extremely important one.[24] Not so long ago some of our more senior colleagues were in the habit of raising the issue of sterilization to young women with MS. Presumably the advice was though kind, and based on an opinion that first, pregnancy can have a detrimental effect on MS, and secondly that a child would be an unfair burden on someone who is likely to become disabled, if they are not already. Nowadays, such advice is generally considered inappropriate. We are better aware of the generally good prognosis for young women with the disease provided they have not shown some of the adverse prognostic indicators described below. Furthermore, there are prospective data which support the general belief that if only young women could be held in a perpetually pregnant state, they would experience no worsening of the disease!.

Results from the 1997 European Pregnancy in MS (PRIMS) study showed a 70% reduction in relapse rate in the last trimester - twice that achievable with the new disease-modifying agents described later. Unfortunately, there is a similar increase in relapse rate in the first three months after delivery. Women with MS who are contemplating a pregnancy can be advised that considering the nine months of gestation plus the three months of the puerperium together, the risk of relapses in that 12 months period is the same as for any other year. If anything, the risk of relapse during pregnancy is a little lower than at other times, but during the first two months post partum the risk is increased, such that the two periods carry the same total risk.

It must be said also that to see a new mother suffer a serious relapse when she is getting used to looking after a baby is particularly hard, and the level of support provided, both physical and psychological, must be at least as good, if not better than, at any other time. The tantalizing observation of a reduced relapse rate later in pregnancy suggests a hormonal influence on the immunological state, which may be to do with a shift in helper T cell populations against the pro-inflammatory cells - this shift reverses after pregnancy, and as yet cannot be maintained.

7.4 Are there any psychological manifestations?

As long ago as 1893, Gowers reported that mood change was a prominent feature in MS, especially an "undue complacency", by which he meant the characteristic elevation of mood, or euphoria, some patients display in the face of disability. It is always difficult to distinguish between the effects of a disease process and a reaction to the fact of the disease, but in comparison with other chronic disabling neurological conditions, there is an increased prevalence of depression in MS patients, as there is in those with predominantly cerebral involvement compared with spinal disease.[25] Regardless of its origin, depression can be a major additional burden for the patient, and needs to be recognized.

As far as cognitive and intellectual functioning is concerned, MS is generally benign causing no more than a relatively minor dissociation between memory function and intellectual ability, though most of us who manage large MS populations can easily list a handful of our patients with clear cognitive and intellectual deterioration. Since they are frequently individuals with extensive disease on MRI and the worst physical disability, there is some measure of comfort to be gleaned from their lack of insight.

Most commonly, intellect is largely retained, but the speed of mental processing may be slowed, as with so many physical functions in MS.

In other words, if they are given enough time, they can perform the task as well as ever. Many patients notice this problem, recognize it as separate from their physical difficulties and can compensate with a little reorganization.

Other recognized psychological disorders associated with MS include "pathological" laughing and crying, cyclothymic swings and emotional hyperexpression.

MULTIPLE SCLEROSIS

CHAPTER 8

THE PROGNOSIS FOR CLINICALLY ISOLATED SYNDROMES AND MS?

8.1 After one attack, what might happen next?

This question commonly arises: the patient has had a single attack suggestive of demyelination and consistent with MS, yet a diagnosis of MS cannot be made since the attack is isolated in both time and space; no dissemination has yet occurred. There are, therefore, two possible outcomes: either the person concerned will, or they will not have further neurological events. If they do, then the diagnosis of MS may be made, depending on the nature and site within the CNS of the attack. If, for example, following on a few months after one attack of optic neuritis, they have a second attack of the same, then the diagnosis of MS cannot be made (incidentally regardless, by convention and by clinical observations of eventual outcome, of whether one or both eyes have been affected by the attacks; the two optic nerves being considered as a single anatomical site), as dissemination in space has not been demonstrated. If, however, the second attack affects eye movements due to a lesion in the brainstem, then the diagnostic criteria for clinically definite MS have been satisfied.

Several epidemiological studies have clarified the risk of developing MS after optic neuritis, but the prognosis for other isolated syndromes, including brainstem attacks and myelitis, is clear well understood. The role of MRI in prognostication after isolated attacks has been discussed in Chapter 5. For optic neuritis, at least 30%, 60% and 70% of affected individuals will develop MS five, 10 and 15 years respectively after this attack. These figures may be slightly lower for other initial attacks, particularly myelitis which, overall, is more likely to be isolated than to lead to MS. Transverse myelitis as an isolated phenomenon is usually more severe initially, but carries a better prognosis for recovery than spinal inflammation as part of MS.

8.2 What are the prognostic indicators for clinically definite MS?

There was a time when physicians were reluctant to discuss the issue of prognosis, telling their patients that it was too variable to given information which was not likely to be misleading. There are enough data now, however, to justify the informed doctor attempting a realistic prognosis. One source of dissatisfaction among patients with MS is the apparent lack of information available to allow them to plan accordingly their lives. Some will continue as if nothing were going to happen, while others will significantly modify their ambitions with respect, for example, to having children, sometimes needlessly.

The most important prognostic factors with respect to future disability have been confirmed by several adequate studies and can form the basis of a discussion with the patient concerning overall prognosis, with the proviso, that MS is notoriously heterogeneous in its outcome and any information given may be inaccurate, occasionally wildly so.[26]

Some of the more valuable indicators of overall clinical prognosis are as follows:

1. Nature of attacks: in general, the more sensory and less motor the attacks, the better the prognosis. In particular, cerebellar involvement, when it appears early augurs poorly for both morbidity and mortality. Brainstem symptoms and sphincter involvement are intermediate in their prognostic importance. If optic neuritis is the first manifestation, then both mortality and morbidity are beneficially influenced. More prolonged attacks are also to be avoided if possible!

2. Interval between attacks: there is conflicting evidence concerning the prognostic value of the interval between the first and second attacks. It was held, somewhat self-evidently that the longer this interval, the better the prognosis, but it now seems that this may not be the case, and that once the disease becomes clinically definite, this interval makes no difference. After the diagnosis is made, however, a higher frequency of attacks generally correlates with a poorer prognosis.

3. Age at onset: all studies have agreed that the younger the age at onset, the better the clinical prognosis. Thus it seems, that what the

young patient loses by developing the disease early, they more than make up for in benign clinical course in the longer term. Conversely, the patient who is diagnosed in their 40s or 50s is likely to experience a more aggressive form of the disease. Taken to the other end of the spectrum is the older patient's tendency to show a primary progressive course from onset (PPMS), where for a given duration of MS, disability is greatest.

4. Recovery from attacks: again rather as would be expected, patients who recover fully from their early attacks show a better prognosis. Those who begin to accumulate fixed disability due to incomplete recover from early attack do less well overall. It has already been stated that an attack that has shown no recovery more than four weeks after onset is likely to recover incompletely if at all.

5. Date of onset: There has been an apparent tendency for the disease to become more benign with the passage of time. Although it has been observed, there is no clear explanation. It appears that patients diagnosed in the 1980s show substantial advantages over those who developed the disease between 1960 and 1979. This observation is independent of duration of disease, and of the use of disease modifying drugs, and seems to apply even more for those diagnosed in the early 1990s.

6. Extent of dissemination: there are clear correlations between prognosis for disability and the extent of dissemination of disease within the CNS. For example the level of fixed disability correlates with whether or not an attack five years before affected a single or multiple neurological systems, the latter heralding a poorer outcome. Similarly, the number of neurological systems affected five years after onset predicts outcome at 15 and 25 years. In general, monosymptomatic attacks and limited dissemination of disease with passing years are more favorable.

7. The brain MRI appearances: as has been described, MRI predicts whether or not an individual who has suffered an isolated attack will ultimately develop the disease. Once MS has been diagnosed, however, the lesion load in the brain is of uncertain predictive value. Some recent studies, performed as part of larger, placebo-controlled treatment trials, have indicated that the lesion load and MRI activity (development of new lesions and contrast-enhancement) over time may correlate with outcome as measured by the EDSS.

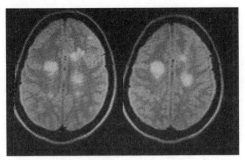

Figure 8.1: The exception that proves the rule? MRI appearances of extensive white matter disease in a patient with benign MS and minimal disability

Formal studies of the relationship between MRI appearances and EDSS have so far failed to confirm a clear relationship, though intuitively one might expect a person with a brain full of white matter lesions to suffer more clinical disability than another with only a small amount, and that a correlation will eventually be confirmed by continuing studies. The exception to this expectation is the case of PPMS in which the degree of disability is usually out of keeping with the minor MRI changes. The explanation for this discrepancy is unclear, but may indicate more diffuse disease beyond the sensitivity of existing MRI techniques, or, more likely, the fact that disability in PPMS is caused by very focal, severe axonal loss, for example in the cervical spine. This latter possibility has received some support from interesting work on this group of patients by Kidd and others that demonstrated marked atrophy of the cervical cord in patients with progressive spastic quadriplegia. Furthermore, similar studies have shown a correlation between the degree of cervical cord atrophy and subsequent clinical prognosis more generally.

In summary, MRI is currently of uncertain value as a prognostic indicator in the established disease, but future work is expected to confirm its usefulness, perhaps by means of specific imaging techniques not yet available in routine studies, which reflect axonal loss within affected pathways.

From these comments it should be clear that, even in the early stages of MS, a pattern of clinical involvement should emerge to allow the experienced clinician to give the patient some notion of what to expect, at least in the short and medium term; it is no longer acceptable to say that the disease is too variable to predict what is likely to happen.

8.3 What is the likelihood of more severe disability or premature death?

Severe disability only affects about one-third of patients overall, with a further third remaining independent in their activities of daily living (ADL) despite moderate disability, and the remaining third suffering mild, minimal or no fixed disability. Half of patients with RRMS will be expected to enter the secondary progressive phase ten years after diagnosis (not onset), and a similar proportion will require some support with walking. It has already been stated that, for a given duration of disease, the primary progressive form of MS carries a worse prognosis for disability.

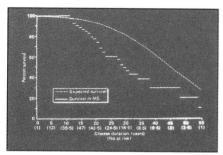

Figure 8.2: Mortality in MS. Kaplan-Meyer plot showing excess mortality from a study of the MS population in New Zealand

Although not a particularly savory topic, many patients do express a wish to discuss their concern that their disease will kill them, and so it is appropriate to discuss it here. Reliable mortality statistics are difficult to obtain in MS, and death certification is notoriously unreliable as a means of determining the true cause of death. Nevertheless, several careful Scandinavian studies have confirmed that there is an excess mortality associated with MS, though it is not great.

Unsurprisingly, the greater the physical disability, the greater the chance of dying of the disease: with an EDSS of seven (unable to walk beyond five meters even with assistance) or greater, there is a 4-fold increase in point mortality at any one time. Conversely, with mild disability (EDSS<3) the relative risk of death is <1.5. The median survival from onset of the disease in men is 28 years (age matched controls 40 years), and for women is 33 years (controls 46 years). The corresponding figures from the time of diagnosis are for men 22 (37) and for women 28 (42) years. Another helpful statistic is that of the excess mortality, which for MS is about 14 per 1000 person-years. The likelihood of dying of an MS-related cause increases with age, and again the dreaded cerebellar involvement is the most prominent clinical manifestation associated with early death. On a brighter note, over the last 20 years there has been a clear trend for excess mortality due to MS to decline, for a variety of reasons including better management of medical complications rather than for a tendency of the disease to become more benign, though this may indeed be the case.

MULTIPLE SCLEROSIS

CHAPTER 9

WHAT CAN BE DONE ABOUT THE SYMPTOMS OF MS?

9.1 Overview

The overall management of a person with MS can be simple or complicated depending on the problems experienced by that person. In the following chapters, the various aspects of management will be described in more detail, including some evolving ideas on how services to support patients with MS and other younger physically disabled people might be organised in the next few years. A number of exciting developments have occurred in the MS field in the last few years, the most prominent of which has been the successful clinical trials of the IFN ß-1a and 1b compounds for first, RRMS, then SPMS.

Other steps forward are no less important though they have received less attention, such as the rapid expansion of a specialist nursing network, and a general increase in people's awareness of the disease and the effort going into fighting it.

The most straightforward aspect of the management of MS is the treatment of individual symptoms by drug therapy and other means.

9.2 What can be done about sensory symptoms?

Sensory symptoms are very common in MS but, fortunately, rarely disabling. Hyperpathia, dysesthesia and paresthesia may be intrusive, and, as they are positive neurological symptoms, may be suppressed by carbamazepine or another anti-epileptic. Decreased sensation including joint position sensation cannot be treated.

9.3 What can be done about motor symptoms?

The motor symptoms which cause the most disability, apart from weakness, about which little can be done, include spasticity, cramps and spasms, tremor and occasionally other abnormal involuntary movements, and eye movement disorders resulting in diplopia, blurring of vision, oscillopsia and just tired eyes.

9.3.1 Spasticity
What is it?

Spasticity, the variable increase in resistance to passive movement characteristic of upper motor neuron disorders causes considerable disability in many patients with MS, but can also be a help to some in maintaining a degree of mobility when otherwise the degree of weakness in their legs would preclude weight-bearing. For this reason, the treatment of spasticity with muscle relaxants must be approached with some care.[27]

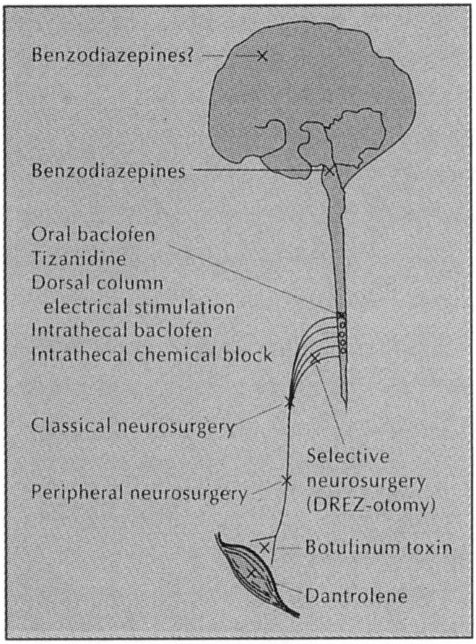

Figure 9.1: The sites of action of the common anti-spasticity agents

Benzodiazepines?
Benzodiazepines
Oral baclofen
Tizanidine
Dorsal column
 electrical stimulation
Intrathecal baclofen
Intrathecal chemical block
Classical neurosurgery
Peripheral neurosurgery
Selective neurosurgery (DREZ-otomy)
Botulinum toxin
Dantrolene

Clinical Assessment

The clinical assessment of the spastic patient with spasticity must be gently conducted as painful spasms might easily be induced by the examination. The various muscles groups are differentially affected; those bearing weight in the legs and the adductors of the hip are particularly important.

Neurological exam and interpretation: Assess for presence of noxious stimuli, which may worsen spasticity, such as UTI, decubitus ulcer, distended bowel and treat. It is most important to remember, however, that there is much more to the proper management of spasticity than just the prescription of muscle relaxing drugs. When such drugs are used, as described below, care is needed to optimize their use, and when more than one drug seems necessary, the sites of action of the different agents should be borne in mind to ensure a logical regimen is prescribed.

Management

The overall management of spasticity is best undertaken with the help of an experienced physiotherapist who can advise the patient on appropriate exercises and, just as important, assess the effect of anti-spasticity medication on mobility.

Oral Medication

The most commonly used agent is Baclofen, a centrally acting agent with potent anti-spasticity activity. It is very important that the initiation of this drug is closely supervised as too rapid a titration may lead to a functionally detrimental loss of muscle tone in the legs. It is also important to ask why the drug is being prescribed and adjust the regimen accordingly. For example, if the principle problem is painful nocturnal spasms then a single bedtime dose is appropriate. If the patient experiences difficulty with walking any distance because the stiffness makes it difficult to swing the leg through and causes premature fatigue, then the correct procedure is to start with a small dose in the morning and instruct the patient gradually to increase it until the desired affect is achieved and the duration of action of the single dose is known. At this point the timing and size of the next dose, if it is required, should be apparent.

It is not recommended to start the patient on multiple daytime doses as these regimens make it difficult to optimize the dosage schedule and carry a greater risk of side effects. Although individual patients' requirements vary enormously, a typical total daily dose would be 20-50mg. Only occasionally do bigger doses confer additional benefit and they are poorly tolerated. As already mentioned, there is also a risk of inducing weakness at higher doses which is counterproductive to mobility. Indeed, it is not uncommon to encounter patients for the first time whose walking is dramatically improved by a reduction in dose and physiotherapy input. The sensible patient will recognize the point at which higher doses begin to make them worse.

Dantrolene is a peripherally-acting muscle relaxant, which is most usefully exhibited as an adjunct to baclofen in patients who require additional muscle relaxation but cannot tolerate higher doses because of drowsiness or increasing weakness. On its own, dantrolene is less useful in MS, and carries a significant risk of hepatotoxicity.

Tizanidine is a new centrally-acting alpha-2 adrenoceptor agonist. Like Baclofen, there is a wide interpatient variability in the effective regimen and dosage. It should be introduced along the same lines, with a gradual dosage titration, preferably in conjunction with the physiotherapists over 4-8 weeks. Maximum effects occur within two hours of taking the drug, usually in an initial dose of four mg, increasing to a usual daily maintenance dose of anywhere between 8 and 36 mg. Up to 80% of patients will notice clinically useful benefit.

The most common adverse effects with tizanidine are drowsiness and a dry mouth. This drug appears not to produce the same degree of counterproductive weakness in the higher dosage range. Physiotherapy supervision is not so crucial but is still desirable.

Nocturnal spasms are often painful and disrupt sleep. Like PTS in MS in general, they are often stimulated by movements during sleep and may, though often do not, respond to traditional remedies like quinine sulphate. If other medication is required, then clonazepam (0.5-2 mg) is usually effective. Diazepam as an anti-spastic is useful in some patients, but many would prefer to avoid diazepam, which is dependency-inducing in the long-term. In some patients who cannot tolerate other agents, however, it may be the best option. In general, the management of spasticity is only partly with drugs; the role of the physiotherapist should not be underestimated.

Implanted Pump

Some people require a higher dose of baclofen for treatment of spasticity, but cannot tolerate the side effects. A surgically implanted pump ('trathecal' baclofen), can administer very small amounts of the drug directly and continuously to the spinal cord (specifically, to an area called the 'intrathecal space'). This technology has been extremely successful for people who have severe spasticity. The baclofen pump may make it easier for people with very limited mobility to be positioned to minimize pain and the risk of skin breakdowns. The pump can improve – or at least maintain – a person's level of daily functioning and it may even help some people remain ambulatory.

The computer–controlled, battery-operated pump, which weighs about six ounces, is surgically implanted under the skin of the abdomen. A tube runs from the pump to the spinal canal. The pump is programmed to release a required dosage of medicine.

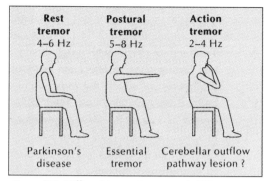

Rest tremor 4–6 Hz	Postural tremor 5–8 Hz	Action tremor 2–4 Hz
Parkinson's disease	Essential tremor	Cerebellar outflow pathway lesion ?

Figure 9.2: Different tremor types seen in MS

People who use the pump return to their physician for a new drug supply and a check of the computer program every one to three months. New drug is injected into the pump through the skin. The small computer can be reprogrammed painlessly by radio signals. When the battery wears out in three to five years, depending on drug dosage, the pump is surgically removed and replaced.

Injections

Botulinum toxin (Botox) injections have been shown to help spasticity. However, the benefit is limited to the injected muscles and the treatment must be repeated very three to six months. Also, only small amounts of the drug can be injected into the body at any one time. Otherwise, the immune system might create antibodies against it.

For these reasons, Botox is not a good choice of treatment when many muscles are spastic or the spastic muscles are large. It is a very good choice when individual muscles are spastic and these muscles are small and do not require a lot of medication. Side effects include weakness of the injected muscle, and, for a few days, some nearby muscles, and a brief, 'flu-like' syndrome. Despite its effectiveness, Botox has not been approved for spasticity in all countries. Another treatment is the injection of a nerve block called Phenol. This treatment also needs to be repeated every three to six months.

Surgical Procedures for more extreme situations

'Rhizotomy' is a surgical procedure in which selected nerve roots are cut at the point where they emerge from the spinal cord. This is sometimes done for the relief of very severe muscle pain. 'Tenotomy', is another surgical procedure, used to correct a joint deformity cased by tendon shortening. It is also used to reduce the imbalance of forces caused by an overactive muscle in a spastic limb.

9.3.2 Speech and swallowing

Disturbances of speech and swallowing are common in MS and when severe, lead to substantial disability and handicap. In the case of swallowing, of course, weight loss and malnutrition can become distressing and eventually life-threatening. However, although very uncommon in MS, the more immediate and potentially life-threatening concern is aspiration pneumonia. Disorders of speech are usually the result either of a pseudobulbar palsy or of cerebellar involvement. Referral to a speech therapy department is often the most expeditious route to helping the patient. Modern aids to communication have rendered almost all suitably motivated patients able to communicate.

Dysphagia, again, is best assessed by the speech, language and swallowing therapists, and sometimes a barium swallow will enable the therapist to advise on the safest posture for eating and optimum consistency of the food. The physician's role is limited. Occasionally a small dose of clonazepam or tizanidine will improve the speech and swallowing of a pseudobulbar patient, but it is not common experience to find the cerebellar patient much better on drugs suggested for tremor (see 9.3.3).

Eventually important decisions must be made with respect to assisted swallowing or the insertion of a percutaneous endoscopically-placed gastrostomy tube (PEG). This decision must be taken in full consultation with the patient, family or carers, and medical attendants, and will depend on the general state of the MS and likely prognosis with and without restoration of adequate food intake. Commonly, of course, such patients are badly disabled overall, but are fully appreciative of the implications, and will make an informed, appropriate decision.

9.3.3 Tremor

Although any clinical type of tremor, including resting tremor, may be seen in MS, the most common and disabling is a manifestation of cerebellar involvement, the intention tremor. This type of tremor characteristically causes oscillation of the limb, which worsens as the target is approached. In the presence of such a tremor, normal muscle strength, postural awareness and cutaneous sensation are useless and cannot compensate. Intention tremor may be focal, affecting a single limb, or more generalized. In the latter case, all voluntary muscle effort is disturbed. Patients may experience wild oscillations of the distal limb endangering themselves and those around them, or find themselves unable to speak comprehensibly due to dramatic variations in the volume of the speech. Even breathing may be affected. Truncal balance may be disturbed to a degree which prevents sitting let alone walking. The tremor may be in one plane, back and forth, which suggests true cerebellar disease, or, in the most disabling cases, multiplanar, sometimes resembling a "bat's wing", in which case the responsible lesion involves the superior cerebellar peduncle or red nucleus.

Management is difficult. For milder tremors, particularly of the arms, isoniazid in high doses (500-1000 mg daily with pyridoxine cover) may suppress it to functional advantage. Alternatively, the anti-epileptics gabapentin and clonazepam are worth a try, and may help some patients. In general though, the appearance of an intention tremor is a "heart-sink" situation and augurs very poorly for the future.

Stereotactic thalamotomy or thalamic stimulation, are procedures that are sometimes considered as a means to help MS patients with tremor. Parkinsonian and essential tremors may respond very well. Its value in cerebellar tremor, however, is less well established, and its efficacy if any, may be temporary. Nevertheless, for selected people with disabling tremor who have failed to respond to medication, a unilateral thalamotomy may confer functional benefit in up to 50% of patients. Bilateral thalamotomies are associated with a high risk of permanent neurological deficit such as dysphasia, and so are no often performed. If being considered for this procedure, patients will usually chose for it to be done on the left to reduce the tremor in their dominant hand. Other measures to reduce intention tremor, such as the use of heavily weighted bracelets, acupuncture and biofeedback are unhelpful.[28]

9.3.4 Oscillopsia and diplopia

Efferent visual disorders such as double vision and environmental movement causes by abnormal involuntary movements of the globes are, fortunately, uncommon as a chronic manifestation of MS. Diplopia due to brainstem disease is usually transient and it is remarkable how the CNS can compensate for continuous movement of the eyeballs as might occur with pendular nystagmus. When they do persist, however, these symptoms are visually disabling and difficult to treat. Diplopia can always be suppressed of course by covering on eye, but stereoscopic vision is abolished by this maneuver.

Oscillopsia will sometimes respond to baclofen and, apparently, gabapentin, though as yet, there are no controlled clinical trails confirming the efficacy of either of these agents. Immobilization of the globes by the injection of botulinum toxin A into the extraocular muscles has occasionally been attempted, but it is remarkably difficult to achieve the desired affect.

9.4 What can be done about paroxysmal symptoms?

As has already been discussed, this category of symptoms is common in MS, and is thought to arise from cross conduction (ephaptic transmission) of impulses between demyelinated, or partially demyelinated fibers. The most common is Lhermitte's symptoms - an unpleasant feeling in the back or limbs or both on flexing the neck. Others include trigeminal neuralgia, PTS and paroxysmal diplopia or dysarthria. There is also an increased incidence of epilepsy in patients with MS compared with the general population.

If treatment is required, these symptoms generally respond well to an anti-epileptic such as carbamazepine. There are several reports in the literature, confirmed by the experience of most clinicians, of the paroxysmal manifestations of MS, even the most powerful and distressing PTS, being suppressed by this drug. A reasonable starting dose, using the slow-release formulation, is 100 mg twice a day initially, increasing gradually. It is disappointing if the relevant symptom is not controlled with 500 mg or less, twice a day. Alternatively, if carbamazepine is ineffective or poorly tolerated, then phenytoin can be prescribed, and gabapentin and lamotrigine are newer agents with similar efficacy, at least anecdotally, though controlled clinical data are, as yet, lacking.

In the specific instance of TGN, if these drugs are unhelpful or side effects are prominent, or even sometimes if the need for them looks like becoming undesirably prolonged, then patients should be advised to consider undergoing one of the trigeminal ganglion lesioning procedures. The skilled operator inserts a needle into the Gasserian ganglion, localizes the spot corresponding to the pain, then freezes, burns or injects phenol depending on preference. In MS, this procedure is very effective and causes little in the way of morbidity, usually in the form of reduced sensation in the relevant part of the face rather than the classical "anesthesia dolorosa". The effects may be permanent, though often it is necessary to repeat the procedure months or years later for recurrent TGN. Drug therapy can often be gradually and successfully withdrawn after the procedure.

It is now generally accepted that, in idiopathic TGN, microvascular decompression of the trigeminal root can be curative. There is some evidence that the efficacy of this procedure is, at least, partially the result of manipulation of the nerve itself. A small number of patients with MS-related TGN have undergone the procedure, usually before the diagnosis became apparent, and it is interesting to note that some have benefited.

9.5 What can be done about bladder, bowel and sexual disorders?

Most disturbances of bladder and bowel function in MS are amenable to successful intervention provided a proper assessment of the problem is carried out first.

9.5.1 Bladder disturbances

It is somewhat artificial to consider bladder problems separate from those of the bowel, since one usually affects the other to some extent. For example, constipation often exacerbates urgency and frequency of micturition, and vice versa, and it is important to bear this in mind when approaching such problems with an intention to treat. As has been described,[20] there are two fundamental bladder disorders in MS; the hyperreflexic bladder causing urgency, urge incontinence, frequency and nocturia in varying proportions, and DSD which involves a combination of hyperreflexic symptoms with difficulty voiding due to coincident impaired sphincter relaxation. As a result the patient notes the uncomfortable sensation of urgency with an inability to empty the bladder briskly or completely. Urgency is experienced by about 80%, frequency by 75%, incontinence by 60%, hesitancy and interrupted stream by 40-50% and incomplete emptying by 35% of patients at some stage in their disease.

While significant difficulties with bladder emptying are easy to recognize, patients are demonstrably unreliable witnesses of early partial retention, and its detection often relies upon proper measurement of bladder emptying, usually in the hospital setting. Indeed, any component of DSD must be recognized and quantified, by means of a post-micturition ultrasound or catheterization of the bladder and measurement of residual urine volume. If this volume is above 100 mls it is indicative, and above 200 mls, diagnostic, of significant retention, and with it, the danger of bladder infection, ureteric dilatation and, eventually serious renal complications. Occasionally, where the situation is less clearcut, referral for a formal urological assessment may be advantageous, and associated with which, urodynamic studies are valuable for guiding management.

Patients with purely hyperreflexic bladders are almost invariably troubled by upper motor neuron symptoms in the legs in MS and indeed any spinal disorder. This association has management implications, since it is surprising how often the patient notices an improvement in bladder function when the leg spasticity is successfully treated. This improvement is only partly explained by a direct effect on bladder wall tone, and it is thought that other spinal mechanisms apply. The correct management of pure hyperreflexic bladder symptoms, which may be so severe as to require the patient to plan his or her life around toilets, depends on a full assessment, including if necessary urodynamic studies.

Provided the level of symptoms is sufficient, the use of bladder relaxants is very effective, and usually restores bladder function to normal, or near normal. The most commonly used agent is oxybutynin, an anticholinergic drug with some specificity for the detrusor muscle, but not free from the usual side effects of such agents, including blurred vision, worsening constipation and a troublesome dry mouth. Other, less specific agents including flavoxate, imipramine and Probanthine are less effective and more prone to produce side effects.

Oxybutynin is prescribed according to the patient's needs. An initial dose is taken at the time of day prior to the most symptomatic period, or as required by planned social activity, and the dose adjusted from 2.5 mg upwards until the symptoms are adequately controlled. Thereafter, further doses are added at not less than four hourly intervals according to requirement. Some patients take it regularly, three or four times daily; others on an 'as and when' necessary basis. Determining the minimum effective dose at the outset is the key to successful treatment. A new agent, tolteridine is now available which offers significant advantages over oxybutynin in terms of tolerability, and probably efficacy, though this latter consideration requires confirmation by continuing clinical trials.

In more severe cases refractory to standard relaxants, more invasive treatments are available in specialist centers. If the bladder has only a very limited storage capacity, then one option is the use of an indwelling suprapubic catheter, which, if properly managed, is a generally safe and satisfactory form of management. Some patients, however, may prefer to consider newer treatments whereby the bladder is either mechanically distended by balloon or more permanently relaxed by the installation of a substance which destroys the delicate neural component of the bladder wall (C-fiber afferents) making it incapable of strong contraction. This treatment is also effective in patients with painful bladder spasms. Capsaicin (basically tobasco sauce), and more recently tolteridine are both effective in this regard, but these treatments are only available in a few centers. They are effective, sometimes for up to six months, and generally well tolerated, so may be repeated, usually with continued success.

Nocturia and enuresis caused by bladder hyperreflexia are distressing symptoms for the sufferer, and may respond to sensible modification of fluid intake with a bedtime dose of oxybutynin or similar. More useful in general, however, is the use of the artificial vasopressin analogue, DDAVP nasal spray, which is taken at bedtime to inhibit urine production overnight. Obviously this treatment is unsuitable if there is renal compromise, and cannot safely be used repeatedly during the 24-hour cycle, but used as a single dose at night is a logical and effective means of alleviating the problem.

9.5.2 Bowel problems

Constipation is the commonest bowel disturbances experienced by MS sufferers. About 45% request treatment for this symptom, though it is surprisingly difficult to manage, perhaps because there are numerous factors which contribute to its development including immobility and drug therapy. Any improvement or removal of aggravating factors is helpful, and a fecal softeners such as lactulose, or and agent like co-danthromer is often somewhat helpful. Fecal urgency and urge incontinence are also common, noted by over 50% of patients in the course of the disease. These are difficult to treat, but may respond to measures that reduce bowel motility, and anticholinergic agents along the lines mentioned above for bladder urgency. Conversely, up to a third of patients with spastic legs and bladder urgency do not have similar bowel symptoms, indicating that they result, to some extent from different neurological mechanisms.

9.5.3 Sexual problems

The sexual problems associated with MS are often untreatable by physical means, though counseling may be very helpful in certain situations. Erectile dysfunction is one exception where, in recent years, advances have been, and are still being made.[29]

MULTIPLE SCLEROSIS

Prior to the introduction of the much publicized sildefanil, there were two different commonly used approaches to the problem, which even now, may still have a place in management of erectile difficulties in men who, for whatever reasons, cannot or will not take this drug. The first is the use of a mechanical vacuum device whereby the penis is made erect by the means of the negative pressure inside a vacuum tube, following which the erection is maintained by applying a constricting rubber ring which exerts pressure above venous but below arterial, the latter for obvious reasons!. The second approach is the intracorporeal injection of a agent such as papaverine or prostaglandin. The former is usually used in doses between ten and 40 mg, or higher in some patients. Prostaglandin E1 is also effective.

There is a natural reluctance among some couples to undertake such injections, and complications, such as priapism occasionally occur. In the longer term, fibrosis may develop, which can cause physical distortion of the penis when erection occurs, a complication very difficult to reverse. On the whole, however, this method is the most effective, though can be labor intensive for those teaching and supervising the technique. It is necessary also to provide round the clock support in case detumescence is delayed as requires withdrawal of blood by syringe.

Yohimbine, extracted from tree bark, was hailed as a genuine aphrodisiac, but was expensive and not particularly effective, and most recently has been developed two valuable treatments, an intraurethral pellet and an oral agent, sildefanil. The latter has been introduced to the market in a spectacular fashion, is effective in the majority of men who take it, but is not free from side effects or abuse potential. Some concerns remain about its use in the more elderly who may not tolerate brisk physical exertions. Some complain of headaches(!) and others of a blue tinge to their vision after taking it.

Other sexual problems including loss of libido and an inability to achieve orgasm may not be related to physical causes and as such, may be amenable to skilled counseling.

9.6 What is available for the dreaded fatigue?

As previously described, fatigue, in its various forms, constitutes one of the most disabling manifestations of MS. There is few weapons available to ameliorate the situation, and common sense advice based on the individual's pattern of fatigue is probably the most useful. For example, it is remarkable how many patients note that they are at their best in the morning and so rush to get everything done by lunchtime. They then feel so tired in the afternoon that nothing can be accomplished. The advice to pace themselves throughout the day often helps considerably. It is important to listen and question carefully about what their fatigue actually constitutes: is it sleepiness, physical exhaustion or aching legs and muscles? All of these forms exist and may be managed separately.

As far as drug therapy for fatigue is concerned, there are a few agents that clearly benefit some patients. First, the mild CNS stimulant pemoline makes a difference in about 50%, and is valuable in this situation. The starting dose is 20 mg taken at the appropriate time of day, but not too close to bedtime because of the side effect of insomnia.

The maximum dose likely to help is 60 mg daily. Unfortunately, because of the tendency of this drug to cause hepatotoxicity in children taking larger doses for hyperactivity, pemoline has been withdrawn from the formulary. It is available, however, on a named-patient basis from the makers, on request, but it is important to monitor liver function before and during treatment.

The alternative is amantadine, the anti-parkinsonian agent. As in idiopathic Parkinson's disease, the mechanism whereby amantadine can help is unclear. The dose is the same as for Parkinson's disease, namely 100 mg daily or twice daily. If there is benefit with these drugs, it is difficult to ascertain whether this is a placebo effect or not, so it is worth considering withdrawal of the drug after six months if there is anything other than a marked response.

A single trial comparing these two drugs came out slightly in favor of amantadine, but the trial did not use full doses of pemoline, and certainly went against most people's expectation.

Most recently, a new agent, modafinil, has become available for excessive daytime somnolescence. Several groups are currently undertaking clinical studies of its potential value for the fatigue associated with MS. Cannabis has been used extensively by patients with MS to alleviate a wide variety of somatic symptoms. Trials are planned in the UK and elsewhere to assess the usefulness of this drug in MS fatigue.

Other drugs, including the stimulant tricyclics, imipramine and clomipramine, occasionally benefit some patients, but in general, fatigue remains a frustrating symptom to treat and a disabling one.

9.7 What can be done about pain syndromes?

The problem of pain, like those of sexual and cognitive disturbances in MS, does not receive the attention it deserves, and should always be questioned after in an assessment.

As described in Chapter 7, the three main types of pain in MS are the neuralgias, myelopathic (spinal) pain, and the chronic musculoskeletal pains. Of course, people with MS are far from immune from all other types of pain that may occur in anyone. Also common are hyperesthesia (reduced pain threshold), dysesthesia (altered pain appreciation) and allodynia whereby different sensory stimuli induce pain. The treatment of the paroxysmal syndromes, including TGN and other neuralgias, has already been described.

The problems concerning myelopathic and other neurogenic pain syndromes are more difficult. In general, the drug of choice is amitriptyline for almost any chronic pain of this type, and indeed this drug is probably the most frequently prescribed agent in the whole of neurological practice. It must be given for long enough and in adequate dose to be effective. I usually commence it in a dose of ten mg an hour before bedtime in all but the strong who can start with 25 mg.

The reason for this caution is that, unlike the case in depression where there is plenty of choice, this agent is very much the best, and it is much more important that the patients get onto the drug than that they do so quickly. The maximum dose likely to help in pain is 50-75 mg, and patients should be warned that the effect is unlikely to be noticeable for at least 2-4 weeks, as the dose is titrated upwards.

The only common side effects of amitriptyline are a dry mouth and sedation. The latter is common even in small doses but tends to diminish quickly. The dose is increased by ten mg a week to the necessary 50 mg or so. It is never helpful to keep going until antidepressant doses are reached, unless depression is also being treated.

This drug will ameliorate almost all of the chronic pain syndromes associated with MS, but some, particularly the more severe burning and stabbing limb pains require more. Carbamazepine again may be helpful, but it is wrong to think that sharp pains are more likely to respond to this drug and dull pains to amitriptyline: as a general rule, both should be tried singly or in combination for patients experiencing a chronic pain syndrome in MS.

Other agents may be helpful in chronic syndromes in MS, and are often worth a try. Mexiletine, an oral analogue of lignocaine, can be strikingly successful in painful diabetic neuropathy, and it may also be worth a try in pain of central origin so long as its use is not cardiologically contraindicated by cardiac conduction defects.

More specialized approaches may require the services of a pain clinic, and include the use of regional and nerve or root blocks or ablations. A lot can be achieved, however, by common sense measures. Neck pain, tension headaches and low back pain can all be helped by a capable and experienced physiotherapist, and transcutaneous nerve stimulation (TENS) and acupuncture in particular are useful in a surprising range of circumstances.

9.8 What can be done about seizures?

When seizures occur as part of an acute attack, and can be differentiated from PTS and other involuntary motor phenomena, they may not require specific treatment, but are found to resolve with the relapse, whether or not steroids are given. If they persist after the relapse has recovered or stabilized for a few months, then if treatment is required on the basis of attack frequency and severity, the usual antiepileptic agents are used, and response is usually satisfactory. Carbamazepine may be appropriate for patients with other paroxysmal manifestations, and the older drugs such as phenobarbitone and phenytoin should be avoided in young adults likely to require long-term therapy. Otherwise, any of the more modern drugs, such as lamotrigine and gabapentin, are acceptable.

9.9 Overview

There is, of course, a wide range of potential symptomatology in a disease such as MS which, by definition may attack any part of the CNS, and it is highly desirable that the provision of services available to the MS sufferer is properly co-ordinated to meet the potential needs of this large group of patients. There is at present a pressing need for the yawning gap between hospital and community-based services to be filed. Several models of care have been proposed, and most would ultimately save money for the purchasers by several mechanisms including a reduction in the need for hospital admission and access to consultants, and the repatriation of monies used to purchase the necessary services elsewhere.

MULTIPLE SCLEROSIS

The best developments of recent years in the field of MS, and one which has been tried and tested in some centers in the USA and elsewhere, is that of nurse-led therapy groups comprising the most important therapists, including physiotherapy, occupational therapy, continence advice and counseling as basic requirements. These groups could be set up in any geographical area with a reasonable population of MS patients. Potential venues for the group might include larger health centers and community hospitals. By this means, the group could provide appropriate therapy in a setting close to the patients' homes, as and when it is required. Such a set-up obviates the difficulties faced by most patients having problems including waiting to see the specialist, then waiting to see the appropriate therapist, by which time the disability is more substantial or the unpleasant crisis is delayed in its resolution.

The role of the specialist MS nurse has become firmly established in the last few years, and many patients have benefited from their input and appreciate their accessibility and expertise. Their general role is in advising on specific areas of management, sometimes including continence advice, and counseling and general support.

With clearly laid out divisions of responsibility, the appointment of a specialist nurse can result in the day-to-day management of patients becoming very much less demanding for the physician, and more efficient in many ways. The nurse tends to empathise with the patients better, and gathers insights into the domestic situation and perhaps underlying problems of a personal or financial nature that the hospital doctor cannot easily address. Supervision is important, especially in the initial stages, but becomes minimal with time, since these girls are usually highly trained. While the advent of the new therapies such as Interferon ß, has brought new hope for patients and raised the profile of MS in recent years, it is still true to say that, the most important component of any MS service remains that which deals with patients' needs quickly and effectively.

CHAPTER 10

WHAT IS THE VALUE OF STEROIDS IN MS?

10.1 Introduction

In clinical practice, the management of relapses in MS has two components; that of the relapse itself, with glucocorticoid (steroid) preparations, and that of the resulting symptoms. It is the first of these components that will be discussed in detail in this chapter. It is important to remember, however, that during a relapse, patients may feel generally unwell and more fatigued.

Supportive care includes rest and the treatment of any precipitating illness, such as a urinary tract infection, which may add to the misery of the relapse. There are theoretical reasons to support the advise to patients to rest during the attack: as discussed in Chapter 3, the acutely inflamed MS lesion associated with relapses may release nitric oxide when axons are activated. This release may contribute to tissue damage. By resting the affected part, therefore, tissue damage may be reduced. Although this hypothesis remains to be tested, it seems reasonable, in the meantime, to advise our patients appropriately.

Despite their almost universal prescription by doctors involved in the management of patients with MS in relapse, there are several important areas of uncertainty in the medical literature concerning the use of steroids. As a result, there is relatively little concordance among doctors with respect to when and to whom steroids should be given, and which regimen to use.

In this chapter, one will find the available information concerning probable mechanisms of action of steroids in MS relapse, efficacy data in different types of disease, and current prescribing habits among neurologists. Finally, some practical guidelines for the use of steroids in MS are proposed.

Multiple Sclerosis

10.2 How do steroids work in MS?

Steroids were first heralded as being of therapeutic value when Hench postulated the existence of "substance X" in 1925, and reported its ability to "cure" rheumatoid arthritis when named cortin in 1949. In those days, Nobel prizes were awarded on the basis of the previous year's events, and it was only in the next couple of years that Hench, having received his, found that the effect was not sustained, and that side effect were significant. The Nobel committee thereafter extended the period of its deliberations!.

It is known, from various lines of evidence, that relapses in MS are associated with immunologically-mediated damage to the blood-brain barrier at an early stage in the evolution of the lesion. Further events, centered on activated T-cells, involve the upregulation and expression of adhesion molecule and cytokine systems, and the recruitment of non-specific T-cells and macrophages.

Glucocorticoids have been shown from experimental and human studies to have wide ranging effects on the immune system, mediated by the type II glucocorticoid receptor. They demarginate neutrophils, raising the peripheral white cell count and induce eosinophil apoptosis (programmed cell death); in macrophages they decrease class II antigen expression, and suppress cytokine, leukotriene and prostaglandin production; they cause a redistribution of T-lymphocytes, induce apoptosis in mature T-cells, and decrease their activation, helper capacity, cytotoxicity and suppression.

Steroids inhibit the production and activity of pro-inflammatory cytokines including some interferons, Il-1, Il-2 and Il-6. They also have a general inhibitory effect on endothelial cell activity, particularly in relation to adhesion molecule expression, including ICAM-1, VCAM-1 and ELAM-1, and adhesion molecule receptor expression on T-cells. Some of these actions, such as T-cell adhesion molecule expression, may not be reflected in serum levels in human disease, and are, therefore, difficult to implicate with certainty in MS relapses. Nevertheless, it is possible to summarize: steroids display potent immunosuppressant activity, which, by a variety of possible (but largely unproven) mechanisms may ameliorate the disease process in MS when in relapse.

Perhaps one of their most important effects in MS is that of stabilization of the damaged BBB. There is considerable MRI evidence to indicate that this effect of steroids on the BBB is at least partly responsible for their beneficial effects in MS relapses, though this can only be part of the story. Gd-enhanced images show an almost complete disappearance of enhancement, which indicates BBB leakage associated with acute lesions, within hours of the first dose. This effect is lost, however, within hours of cessation of the steroid treatment. This effect of steroids cannot, therefore be the sole mechanism whereby they bring about recovery from relapses, as is also indicated by the observation that longer steroid courses (for example, three weeks) are not significantly more effective than shorter (three days) ones.

10.3 What is the clinical efficacy of steroids in MS relapses?

The clearest way of summarizing the usefulness of steroids in the context of MS is to say that they have been shown to shorten the recovery time of relapses in MS, but they do not appear usually to influence the ultimate degree of recovery, nor do they have any influence on the longer term natural history of the disease.

The first form of steroid therapy to enjoy widespread use in MS was adrenocorticotrophic hormone (ACTH). The problem with the ACTH form of steroid therapy was that it caused unselected release of steroids from the adrenals in unpredictable quantities. Unfortunately, at the time there were no good data on the efficacy of ACTH to justify its use or to compare it with other forms of steroids.

Gradually, however, studies were published which first suggested at, then proved the efficacy of steroids in hastening recovery from relapse. By the 1970s, steroids became an accepted form of treatment in MS, and over the next 20 years, first clinical, then MRI data emerged confirming their efficacy and suggesting that at least some of the possible mechanisms of action already discussed may be important.

Several studies have demonstrated the superiority of steroids compared to placebo in shortening recovery in relapses, though the best regimens to use remain unclear. In one of the first controlled trials of ACTH in the treatment of relapse, significant improvement by the end of the three week trial period was found in 11 of 22 treated patients compared with four of 18 in the control group, a result reproduced by a similar study of 197 MS patients. In the latter trial, at each time interval, more treated patients improved significantly, the largest difference being observed at two weeks, with 57% versus 38% of treated and control patients respectively improving, and at four weeks, with figures of 65% versus 48%.

By the mid-1980s, the general perception of steroids in MS was that ACTH was less predictable and no more effective than other regimens and so was dropped from general usage. To take its place, intravenous methylprednisolone (IVMP) was shown in trials to be at least as effective. One trial at least compared directly the efficacy of ACTH and IVMP, and was unable to demonstrate a difference between the two treatment groups.[30]

More recently, various low and high-dose oral steroids regimens have been the subject of numerous reports as being less expensive, more convenient, and probably safer in terms of side effects than IVMP.[31] The most recent, from Denmark, describes a randomized study of 25 patients in relapse treated with placebo compared with 26 treated with oral methylprednisolone, 500 mg for five days followed by a ten day oral taper. Their results strongly favor the treated group by several measures over an eight week period. How oral and IVMP compare in efficacy is probably still not fully established. Alam et al compared identical doses (500 mg a day for five consecutive days) of oral MP and IVMP in small groups of patients, and was unable to show any differences between them.[32] Nevertheless, there remained, and indeed remains an intuitive impression among neurologists that the IVMP regimens somehow better.

In a attempt to test this hypothesis, Barnes et al, in 1997 described a study of 80 patients treated with either IVMP (1 gm for five days) or OMP (48 mg for seven days; 24 mg for seven days and 12 mg for seven days), in which several outcome measures were used, none of which showed any significant benefit of either regimen.[34]

While it has been possible to level criticism at many, particularly the earlier, of these studies, none have been able to demonstrate any longer-term implications for the use of steroids in MS relapses, in terms of improving the outcome of relapses or long-term disability. The same cannot be said for the studies of optic neuritis, however.

With the publication of the optic neuritis treatment trial in 1992, came the suggestion that, even allowing for pre-study difference in MRI appearances, patients treated with low-dose oral prednisone seemed to have a greater likelihood of going on to develop clinically definite MS at six months.[33] This observation, though not an original endpoint of the study did carry conviction, and many clinicians, particularly in Canada and the USA significantly modified their steroid prescribing in MS. With the later publication of the three year follow-up data, however, any observed difference seemed to have disappeared, and the concern associated with low-dose steroids in MS diminished, though probably has not altogether gone. Other studies of optic neuritis have suggested that in some subgroups, steroids may beneficially affect eventual recovery. Those patients with longer lesions on MRI, and those with intra-canalicular MRI disease seem to do worst, and steroids probably improve eventual visual outcome, though these patients are difficult to distinguish clinically.

To sumarize the evidence concerning the use of steroids in relapses of MS: they are effective in hastening recovery from clinical relapse, but do not usually benefit eventual outcome, either in terms of degree of recovery or subsequent disease activity. In certain patients with optic neuritis, however, recovery may be improved by steroids. Which type and regimen to use is undecided, but there is good evidence to show that both oral and IV regimens are effective, and no controlled data showing superiority of one over the other in any dosage in MS. Again, however, optic neuritis, when isolated, seems more responsive to higher rather than lower dose regimens.

10.4 What is the role of steroids in progressive MS?

While it is now common practice to use steroids for MS relapses, the situation in other types of MS is not well documented, and trials are needed: there are no proper data of the treatment of progressive MS with continuous steroid therapy over years. Steroids are not usually indicated, therefore, for either primary or secondary progressive MS as they are of no proven benefit, and are potentially harmful in the long-term. Any consideration of longer term steroid use in MS is inappropriate in our present state of knowledge. In other words, the potential risks outweigh the potential benefits

The only exception to this rule is the very occasional patient with true steroid-dependency, in whom withdrawal leads to an objective neurological deterioration (not just a feeling of unwellness). Such patients are uncommon, and indeed it may be difficult to be sure that some other process such as sarcoidosis or a vasculitis is not responsible.

Having stated that in our present state of knowledge, long-term steroids currently have no place in the management of MS, many clinicians feel that no patient with progressive neurological disability due to MS should been allowed to worsen without at least once being given a course of steroids: occasionally the response is worthwhile, and the risk is minimal. It is not always easy to make a judgement on the pattern of the disease, and some patients who appear to be progressing, are, in fact, having relapses. It is these patients that need to be identified, and lend justification to the policy, not universally held, of giving steroids at least once to every MS sufferer.

It has been suggested by a few studies that some patients with secondary progressive MS do seem clearly to benefit from a three or four monthly course of oral prednisolone, even though in general steroids are not used in progressive MS of any kind unless there is a superimposed relapse of sufficient severity to justify their prescription. This policy is supported by the sparse literature available on the subject which suggests that in the short term there may be benefit, particularly in pyramidal function from regular steroid courses.

10.5 What is the current practice of clinical neurologists using steroids in MS?

It is clear that the majority of relapses in MS patients never come to the attention of the specialist. Many patients simply do not mention less severe attacks, or they contact their GPs who may give them an oral course of steroids without reference to the local neurologist. It is unknown, therefore, exactly to whom, in what form, and how frequently steroids are actually given in MS. However, in these days of evidence-based medicine, it is important to understand the current situation among specialists in a field to determine the extent to which such evidence as exists is incorporated into clinical practice, and to identify those areas where more evidence is clearly needed.

To this end, two recent surveys of UK neurologists have been carried out. The first by a group in Cardiff, and the second in London. The results of these surveys can be sumarized as follows:

Nearly all respondents agreed that steroids are effective in shortening recovery from relapses, but erred on the side of disagreement with the suggestion that they may improve the eventual outcome of a relapse. About 80% prescribe steroids in more than a quarter of all relapses, but less than 5% never use steroids. More than 50% always, and 99% at least sometimes use IVMP as the steroid of first choice. Conversely only 5% use oral steroids as first choice routinely, and 70% rarely if ever use oral steroids in MS. Curiously, there was an even split when the question of superior efficacy of IVMP over oral came up: presumably, the continued preference for IVMP indicates in part a feeling that IV should be better, in part a lack of conviction concerning the available comparative data, and in part, habit. In was interesting to note that, despite our finding of no significant difference between oral and IV steroid efficacy, there had been no significant change in the proportion of courses given as each between 1996 and 1998, the paper having been published in 1997.

There is little evidence of fixed policies where steroid prescribing is concerned; only 20% admitting to always following one. The dosages and regimens of IVMP used varied considerably from 250 mg to 1000 mg daily for anything from two to five days, the most common being one gm daily for three days, or 0.5 gm daily for five days. Very few UK neurologists, however, give an oral taper. It appears that very few patients refuse the offer of steroids, and that admission to hospital solely to give IVMP is becoming less popular, though about a third do so at least some of the time. Conversely, the majority of IVMP courses are administered to inpatients, so presumably, these patients have the worst attacks, justifying admission on their own.

When oral steroids are used, prednisolone is the preferred agent, though some routinely use oral dexamethasone or methylprednisolone. The last of these probably has the best claim to usage if the recently published report of its very clear superiority (in high dose) over placebo is correct. In this study, the actively treated patients did significantly better at one, three and eight weeks after initiation of treatment, according to a number of measures including the EDSS and Scripps neurological rating scale.[7]

The majority of neurologists indicated that they try to limit the number of courses any one patient receives in a given 12

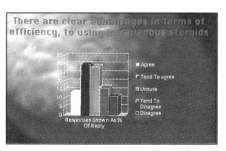

Figure 10.1a: Steroids are not used as long-term management for MS

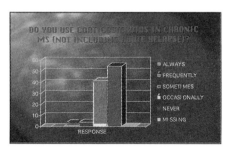

Figure 10.1b: Steroids are not used as long-term management for MS

month period. This presumably reflects the very real concern over cumulative side effects of steroids. The majority of neurologists disagree, or tend to disagree with the routine prescription of steroids in MS by GPs, though a significant minority had no such objection. Most were in the habit of reviewing the outcome of a course of steroids given for MS relapse.

Respondents were almost unanimous that, in our current state of knowledge, there is no place for long-term steroid use in MS. Nearly a quarter, however, felt that there was a place for steroids in MS other than for relapse. A separate question asked whether every patient with MS should have at least one course of steroids to assess responsiveness, a suggestion with which most just over half disagreed. Experience was mixed with respect to truly steroid-dependent patients with MS, only a small majority favoring their existence.

10.6 How should steroids be given for MS relapses?

When considering which relapses should be treated with steroids (should the patient chose to take them), it is not particularly important to consider how often they have been given in the past. In general, however, it is sensible to limit the number of courses, if possible, to three a year, though there are no good data to say that more are harmful in the long-term, and IVMP courses are not clearly associated with a reduction in bone density. Some patients may require more to be optimally treated, but is not good practice to prescribe steroids indiscriminately for MS relapses; the decision should be at least partly dictated by the severity of the attack, and by the amount of disability and handicap it produces. What will be disabling for one individual may only be an inconvenience for another, and non-disabling attacks will almost always recover satisfactorily without treatment.

Another consideration will be the type of attack: while in general it is thought that steroids do not influence outcome, some attacks may do better after steroids. For example, severe optic neuritis with complete visual loss is sometimes caused by an unusually long lesion in the optic nerve, or by involvement of the nerve in the bony canal. Here, steroids may improve outcome and should be considered. Another example is an attack affecting cerebellar function. Ataxia and dysmetria are among the most disabling manifestations of MS, and fixed disability of this type carries a very poor long-term prognosis. Steroids should be considered for any attack that causes significant cerebellar damage. These considerations are, to some extent, based on personal experience and preference, but in the absence of hard data, we must take decisions in the best interests of our patients.

As far as which type of steroid, and in what dose, there is little or no concensus either within or between countries, mainly due to lack of comparative efficacy data. Surveys indicate that in the UK at least, the most popular regimens for IV and oral steroids respectively include:

IVMP 1gm daily for three days or 0.5 gm for five days.

Oral prednisolone tapering from 60 mg over about three weeks, for example 60, 45, 30, 15 and 5 mg each for five days. (There is evidence from at least two controlled trials to justify the routine prescription by some of high-dose oral methylprednisolone, for example 500 mg for five days, as recommended by Sellebjerg et al[35]).

As yet, the use of an oral taper remains a matter of personal preference: they are more popular in the USA, but less so in Europe, and higher doses and longer courses of both IV and oral steroids are not uncommonly prescribed.

At present, therefore, the listed regimens, or minor modifications of them, remain standard in most parts of the world, and significant changes must be introduced on the basis of proper controlled and randomized trials demonstrating significant benefit.

10.7 Summary

In summary, there is clear evidence to support the use of steroids in relapses of MS, since they hasten recovery, though do not, in general, improve eventual outcome. There are no generally agreed protocols with respect to which type of steroid, or how much to give, though most clinicians use high-dose IVMP as first choice. A minority use oral prednisolone, though recent evidence supports the prescription of higher dose methylprednisolone as the oral steroid of first choice.

Relapses should be treated on their merits with a decision being taken on the basis of relapse severity and type, and the amount of disability and handicap it produces in that individual. There is no place for the indiscriminate use of steroids for all relapses; indeed probably no more than 10-20% of all relapses merit their use.

With respect to progressive MS, there is no evidence to support the use of steroids in these groups of patients, but if there is any doubt about the pattern of disease in a deteriorating patient, it is not unreasonable to recommend that steroids be tried at least once, as the risk is small. There is also a lack of evidence concerning the long-term use of steroids in MS, and they are not used in this way except in the rare patient with true steroid-dependency. Some evidence exists to suggest that oral pulses may be of benefit in secondary progressive MS in the medium term.

Much further work could be done to advantage in this field, but it is unlikely that too many individuals will be enthusiastic, particularly with the emergence of more compounds with the potential to affect beneficially the natural history of this disease. Nevertheless, steroids have underpinned our management of MS attacks for the last three decades and more and should still be considered a useful weapon in the fight against MS.

CHAPTER 11

CAN ANYTHING MAKE A DIFFERENCE TO THE NATURAL HISTORY OF MS?

11.1 What should I know about Interferon ß preparations?

The introduction of Interferon ß in the management of MS has provided real hope that the natural history of the disease can be modified to the benefit of the patient. After a false start with Interferon γ, which was found to increase the rate of relapses in RRMS (but which provided some useful lessons and pointers along the way), considerable interest was generated by results with Interferon ß in the 1980s and early 1990s. This culminated in the publication, in 1993, of the "pivotal" paper on the clinical results of the first large, randomized, placebo-controlled trial with interferon ß in RRMS.[36] The subsequent introduction of Interferon b into clinical practice has raised the profile of MS in both the public and political arenas over the last few years. There is now clinical experience available on several 100,000 patient-years with this agent, in terms of its safely, tolerability and efficacy.

For the first time, there is clear evidence that a treatment may safely and beneficially influence the natural history of both RR and SPMS. Interferon-ß is successful in suppressing relapses in RRMS and delaying progression of the disease, although the effect on these parameters in all patients is not as great as could be hoped. Nevertheless, in selected patients, the reduction in relapse rate by about a third is valuable. In addition, a slowing of progression of disability may, in most patients, be regarded as the more important reason for considering treatment with this agent.

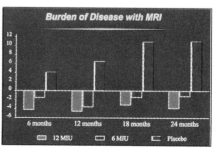

Figure 11.1: MRI confirms a marked reduction in disease activity, which is dose related

MULTIPLE SCLEROSIS

The first major clinical trial of interferon ß in RRMS used interferon ß-1b. The primary endpoints were the annual relapse rate and the proportion of patients remaining relapse-free: the secondary endpoints were the time to first relapse, relapse duration and severity, change in EDSS from baseline, disease burden on annual MRI scans and disease activity on serial scanning. The results were received with mixed feelings, and no little cynicism, though the majority felt that the MRI data in particular were promising, and the overall impression was favorable. Many, but far from all, neurologists felt that this drug should be made available to their patients with RRMS who fulfilled the clinical criteria laid down by the trial.

In the USA, interferon ß-1b received its license and, predictably, to date over 30,000 patients, representing about 10% of the MS population, have been put on the drug. The politics of the situation, as much as anything, meant that after approval was granted in early 1996, less than 2% of all MS patients, about 1,000 in all, went onto treatment. This was not universally the case in Europe however, where, overall, 6% (20,000 patients) have received treatment to date. Germany and Greece, in particular, approached the 10% mark for the proportion of their whole MS population put on the drug.

The publication, in 1996, of the results of the first major study with interferon ß-1a (identical to human interferon) in RRMS was greeted with considerable enthusiasm.[37] The reduction in relapse rate reported in this study was somewhat lower than with interferon ß-1b, although this could be plausibly attributed to the lower dosage of interferon. Even though the specific activity of interferon ß-1a is some 10-15 fold greater than that of interferon ß-1b,38 the dose of 30 mcg once weekly (given by intramuscular injection) was considerably lower than the standard dose of interferon ß-1b of 250 mcg every alternate day. It was also claimed that treatment with interferon ß-1a substantially slowed the progression of disability. However, as this study included only patients who were impaired rather than disabled, and the subgroup of 57% patients who completed the full two years of the study contributed disproportionately to the outcome, not all physicians were persuaded by this disability claim.

In 1997, the situation changed when the PRISMS data were announced.[39] In this study, interferon ß-1a was given subcutaneously (SC) at a dose of 22 mcg or 44 mcg three times a week for two years to patients with RRMS. The results confirmed beyond reasonable doubt that interferon ß, when given at a sufficient dose, is effective in suppressing both the relapse rate and severity, and also in slowing progression of disability in RRMS.

It is important to remember, however, that there are still very few data concerning treatments to modify the natural history of MS beyond three years. A recent study of sulphasalazine showed that after an initial improvement, patients on active treatment seemed to regress after three years. The lesson is clear: whilst therapy with interferon ß, glatiramer acetate and other undoubtedly offers hope in MS, the situation with respect to long-term response and benefit remains quite unproven until further data become available, if ever such trial are done.

At the time of writing, three interferon ß products are available and licensed for this form of the disease: one is interferon ß-1b and two are interferon ß-1a molecules, the latter being chemically identical to the interferon ß produced in our own bodies.

11.2 Who is Suitable for Treatment with Interferon ß?

The clinical criteria for therapy with interferon ß to be applied to potential candidates with RRMS were derived from the original pivotal study of interferon ß-1b. They were agreed with reasonable accord throughout Europe, and individually within the USA. These criteria were designed originally for trial use, but were applied subsequently in clinical practice. Unusually, the matter was considered of sufficient importance by the UK government that an executive letter, EL(95)[97], was issued on the subject in November 1995. In this document it was stated that "...and in particular, *to initiate and continue prescribing of Beta-Interferon through hospitals.*" Although the clinical criteria are specific, they should be regarded as guidelines and be applied intelligently, and with the best interests of the individual concerned at heart. The criteria were:

- Age over 18 and preferably under 55;

- Clinically definite RRMS, but no evidence of progression;

- Ambulant without aid or rest for 100 meters (EDSS 5.5 or better);

- Disease activity to justify therapy - at least two relapses in the past two years severe enough to justify steroid therapy in the opinion of the physician;

- No other medical problems contraindicating the use of interferon ß.

MULTIPLE SCLEROSIS

It can be appreciated from this list of criteria, that a certain amount of common sense is required on the part of both the clinician and the patient. Clearly, if a patient is suitable in all ways, but cannot manage to walk the 100 meter distance for some other reason, such as an amputation, it would be wholly unreasonable to withhold treatment. The principle, of course, is that a patient who is already very disabled does not come out on top of the risks, benefits equation.

The really difficult issue, however, is that of disease activity. We have experienced major problems in deciding how to advise some patients in this regard. Broadly speaking, the most suitable patients for Interferon ß therapy are those with frequent attacks, those with unnervingly unpleasant attacks (such as repeated cerebellar or brainstem episodes), and those in whom attacks generally seem to recover incompletely.

In the light of new findings, however, recommendations on when treatment should commence may be reconsidered in the near future. A recent pathological study has shown that axonal damage and loss is a consistent feature of chronic MS, as described in Chapter 3. This irreversible form of damage may even begin very early in the course of the disease.[40] Thus, early treatment with interferon ß may be necessary to obtain optimal protection of axons. The potential importance of these findings is reflected in a recent consensus statement from the US National Multiple Sclerosis Society which recommends that "initiation of therapy is advised as soon as possible following a definite diagnosis of MS and determination of a relapsing course."[41] We await with interest the results of on-going clinical trials with Interferon ß given in early MS, which should clarify this situation and may alter our prescribing practice. In the meantime, however, we must remain objective and consistent in our evidence-based practice.

Not every patient with RRMS will automatically want to go onto treatment with interferon ß. The most common reason we have found for refusal of treatment in an otherwise suitable candidate has been a benign pattern of attacks, even though these may be quite frequent in some patients. Several such people have decided to 'wait and see' on the grounds that attacks are always sensory and stereotyped and recover fully and quickly. Others are clearly following a benign course, despite continuing attacks, and decide to wait.

If a patient fulfils the criteria, it is up to him or her, when in possession of all the relevant facts, to decide whether or not it is the right time to begin treatment. Many choose to wait, and others require more time to think about it, as this decision is not to be rushed given the implications in terms of time and effort on the part of both the patient and clinician, and the potential for side effects. Most people, however, are sufficiently informed prior to the clinical assessment to have reached a decision to accept if treatment is offered. We have also found that very few people are upset by a refusal once the situation has been explained clearly and sympathetically.

11.3 How is Interferon ß prescribed, and administered, and what are the problems?

Prescribing of these drugs is by specialists, usually neurologists. In the UK, at least, general practitioners have not been encouraged, and have been understandably reluctant, to get involved with the actual decision-making process and prescription of the drugs.

Having gone through the assessment stage and been offered treatment with interferon ß, patients will next be seen and given instructions by the specialist nurse, sometimes with the help of videos and always with written material. It is explained that all three of the interferon ß preparations are given by injection, one intramuscularly, the other two subcutaneously. We have found that only a very small number of people have difficulty with the injections, which are usually self-administered, although some rely on a carer or nurse for reasons of disability or nervousness. The problems encountered can be reduced significantly by proper instruction in injection technique, and clear explanation and demonstration. In the various clinical trials, the usual dropout rate as a direct result of side effects of interferon ß has been very low, at less than 5% with interferon ß-1a and 8% with interferon ß-1b.

In the first few weeks or months, injection site reactions are experienced by at least two-thirds of patients using the subcutaneous (SC) formulations, but usually consist of no more than transient redness and minor swelling at the injection site. About 5% of patients experience more discomfort or prolonged reactions, with induration and discoloration being persistent and unsightly, or the development of skin necrosis. These problems may be at least partially obviated by adjusting the injection technique. For example the routine use of a two needle technique, whereby a fresh needle is used after drawing up the liquid, removes the risk of a needle track reaction. Such a procedure is, however, unnecessary with the most recent interferon ß-1a preparation, which is supplied in liquid pre-filled syringes for immediate SC injection. Also, for some reason, injection into the buttock seems to be much better tolerated than injection elsewhere. Only two of our patients have discontinued treatment, despite counseling, because of persistent troublesome skin problems.

The other common initial problem is a 'flu-like reaction which tends to appear within a few hours of the injections. Some 52-61% of patients get this symptom, but it is rarely incapacitating. Patients need to be warned of its occurrence and advised to take their injections last thing at night so that the reaction has passed by the time they get up next morning. If it is troublesome, its severity can be reduced by taking diclofenac, or a similar preparation, before the injection can reduce its severity.

In addition to these most common problems, others include (approximate percentage of patients more than placebo) increased liver enzymes (25); lymphopenia (9); myalgia (15); fever (9), and a few other minor symptoms. More importantly, and despite anticipation to the contrary, depression, or worsening of pre-existing depression with suicide risk, clinically significant lymphopenia or liver toxicity, or any other important adverse events, did not appear as problems.

The key to the successful and trouble-free introduction of interferon ß therapy is presence of the specialist nurse. When interferon ß-1b was first introduced in the USA and Europe, a network of support nurses with special training in its use, and in MS more generally, was also provided. Without these nurses, it would be quite impossible to provide the information and training the patients require initially, and the continued support they all seek and need subsequently. Indeed, it would be no more possible to provide treatment with interferon ß in the UK without the nurses than without the needles and syringes.

11.4 Which Interferon ß should we use?

The short answer is that it is up to the patient to choose, having been appraised of the relative benefits and drawbacks of each of the three available preparations. In practice, of course, they will often ask which is the best choice; which would the physician take?

To date, no formal comparisons of the different interferon ß preparations have been undertaken. Where any comparison is concerned, therefore, it must be remembered that the various trials were carried out to different designs, with different patient populations and different clinical endpoints.

Endpoint Weekly dose	ß-1a (SC)		ß-1a (IM) 30 mcg	ß-1b (SC) 875 mcg
	66 mcg	132 mcg		
Reduction in relapse rate, 2 years (%)	29	32	18* (32)	31† (34)
Increase in relapse-free patients at 2 years (%)	69	119	46	56‡ (94)
Increase in time to first relapse (%)	70	113	31	93
Reduction in mod/severe relapses (%)	28	37	18* (32)	49
Reduction in hospital admissions (%)	21	48	not stated	36
Reduction of disease activity on MRI (%)**	67	78	33	79#

* All patients treated using all time in the study (post hoc analysis of subset of patients followed for 2 years). This study included only moderate/severe relapses.
† All patients value (published value relating to data from 338 of the 372 patients).
‡ Value based on data in FDA package insert (published data).
# approximate figure from data available.
** Data are not directly comparable because the three studies use different measures of MRI activity.

Table 11.1 Comparison of main trial endpoints for each of the three Interferon ß products.

These limitations notwithstanding, the results of the three trials confirm the efficacy of interferon ß in RRMS, and their findings are sumarized in Table 11.1.

In addition to the data given in Table 11.1 in relation to relapses, there were arguably more important data concerning progression of disability. The pivotal study of interferon ß-1b in RRMS was not designed to show an effect on disability, although despite this, to its credit, it did hint at a trend in favor of active treatment (Table 11.2). Although the first interferon ß-1a data purported to show benefit, the figures on such an important issue were thought by most experts to require confirmation before they could be used as a basis for making management decisions. Such confirmation became available, and further valuable data were added by the PRISMS data for interferon ß-1a became available.

PRISMS was the first study to show consistent efficacy with interferon ß in all major endpoints, and provided persuasive evidence of a positive effect with respect to the time taken to reach a measurable, sustained worsening of disability. Unfortunately, through no fault of the investigators, all of these carefully (and expensively) gathered pieces of trial data are marred to some extent by the very inadequate tools by which disability has necessarily had to be measured (the EDSS in particular lacks sensitivity and specificity). Even allowing for these imperfections, the data showed that, with interferon ß-1a, the time to confirmed progression of disability was significantly prolonged. Indeed, PRISMS showed a 55% and 79% improvement with 22mcg and 44mcg respectively.

EDSS change	Worse	Stable	Improved
Interferon ß-1a (IM) Subgroup of 111 patients with EDSS 1-3.5 who completed two years on the study; EDSS change confirmed			
Treated	18.2%	63.6%	18.2%
Placebo	30.3%	60.7%	8.9%
Interferon ß-1b – Patients with EDSS up to 5.5; EDSS change confirmed			
8 MIU	20%	80%	NA
1.6MIU	28%	72%	NA
Placebo	28%	72%	NA

Table 11.2 Percentages of patients receiving interferon ß-1a (IM), interferon ß-1b, or placebo, whose EDSS score worsened, improved or remained stable after treatment

So, with these data available, and now having eight years' or more experience with these compounds in the USA and five years' in Europe, which is the best type of interferon ß for our patients?

The main difference in practical use is that one of the interferon ß-1a compounds is given three times weekly by SC injection, and the other weekly by intramuscular (IM) injection, whereas interferon ß-1b is given SC on alternate days. The availability of the most recent interferon ß-1a product in liquid pre-filled syringes for SC injection makes the three times weekly administration procedure considerably easier for the patient. It is also the general impression that the once-weekly IM injection of interferon ß-1a can be painful, but this route does produce less in the way of troublesome skin reactions. In practice, these considerations do not seem to influence patients to any great extent.

A recent study has shown that there is no significant difference in the severity or duration of side effects with interferon ß-1a given IM once weekly compared with interferon ß-1b given SC every alternate day.[42] In any case, the common side-effect of 'flu-like symptoms tends to diminish or disappear altogether within a few weeks or months, and is rarely very troublesome. Generally, indeed, all three interferons are very well tolerated with only small numbers of patients discontinuing therapy because of side effects.

On the face of it, when comparing the two interferon ß-1a preparations, there appears to be an important cost-benefit consideration. Given that the SC and IM preparations contain the same active compound, but in different formulations, then by virtue of the chosen trial dosage regimens, SC interferon ß-1a provides twice as much of the active substance than IM interferon ß-1a for the same amount of money. It has, however, been suggested that the bioavailability of IM is better than SC interferon. This was based on a study that included 16 volunteers but did not have a cross-over design.[43]

A more recent cross-over study in 30 volunteers has shown the two products to be bioequivalent according to FDA guidelines, despite the different routes of administration.[44] Optimum dosage and route of administration remain unresolved, though intuitively it seems likely that, within limits, a larger dose is likely to be to be more effective, and evidence is accumulating to support this view.[45, 46]

From a practical viewpoint, it is often the preparation with which the doctor is most familiar which is the most acceptable. What evidence exists favors a higher rather than lower dose, and there are those who favor SC over IM injections and vice versa. The frequency of injection can also be viewed from two perspectives: some feel that a more frequent injection "must be doing me more good". The patient who is already doing well on a preparation should be treated according to the "if it ain't broken, don't fix it!" principle.

For patients being considered for treatment for the first time, their choice is between the greater familiarity with interferon ß-1b versus the theoretical advantages of the natural human substance; between the single weekly, but potentially painful IM and more frequent but easier and more gentle SC injection. Switching from one preparation to another because of perceived lack of efficacy is unlikely to be a useful strategy unless the patient has developed a high level of neutralizing antibodies (NAB) on 1b as described in the next section. Similarly, the side-effect profile of each preparation is almost identical!

11.5 What is the relevance of neutralizing antibodies?

There is another issue that may influence the initial choice of interferon ß or the subsequent decision to switch a patient from one to another interferon ß preparation, and that is the development of neutralizing antibodies. Some 38% of those on interferon ß-1b will develop NAB in their serum, whereas the figure for interferon ß-1a is 18-22% in significant titres (>20). It is unlikely that there is any important difference between IM and SC interferon ß-1a in terms of NAB development, but the higher risk with 1b is probably explained by its chemical differences from the human compound.

Because the interferon ß molecules are potentially antigenic, it is not surprising that some patients will develop NAB when exposed to them. Intuitively, it seems likely that if a patient develops a high NAB titre in their serum, then the effect of the interferon ß they are taking will be diminished or lost altogether. There is some evidence for this conclusion from long-term efficacy data, particularly with respect to interferon ß-1b, which differs in molecular structure from the natural molecule, is unglycosylated, and is more antigenic than the interferon ß-1a preparations.

The clinical significance of NAB-positive status is, however, unproven: a reanalysis of the data pertaining to interferon ß-1b apparently showed that the loss of clinical efficacy was only significant for the lower drug dose, and that those developing NAB may lose them from the serum later, or the titer drops significantly. There have even been suggestions that the development of NAB might increase the drug's beneficial effect on disability, though this is difficult to believe, and even harder to prove convincingly.

In summary, the importance of NAB remains unknown, there being no evidence positively demonstrating their clinical importance in patients taking standard doses of interferon ß, either 1a or 1b. Anecdotal evidence does, however, indicate that very high titer of NAB (>640), as found in a few patients on 1b (9 out of 40 patients in one unpublished series), are relevant, and likely to lead to a diminution of response.

One practical policy, therefore, is to test for NAB at 12 months, and to consider a switch from 1b to 1a if levels are very high (after which 50% lose the NAB after 6 months), or switch to 1b or discontinue therapy if on 1a. Lower positive levels can be remeasured after 6 months, at which time they may have fallen or disappeared, in which case therapy is continued unchanged; if they have risen to very high levels then the above policy applies. It should be reiterated, however, that at the moment there are no firm data to support the use of NAB in clinical decision-making, and many clinicians will prefer to advise their patients on grounds of clinical responsiveness.

11.6 What is the situation with respect to PP and SPMS?

There are currently no data on the usefulness or otherwise of these compounds in PPMS, though at least one trial is underway. It seems unlikely, however, that it will be possible to demonstrate a positive effect in this form of MS, though the trials may surprise us yet.

We do, however, have some data on the use of interferon ß-1b in SPMS in a study involving over 700 patients, and comparing the standard dose of interferon ß-1b with placebo, for what was initially planned as a 3-year trial.[47] An interim analysis proved positive, however, and so the trial was terminated with data available for a mean of almost 2.5 years, with 74% of patients either still being treated at interim cut-off or having completed the full three years of treatment. The primary endpoint was the time to sustained progression of disability by one EDSS point. The results showed that, at 16-18 months, 40% of the placebo group had progressed compared to only 27% in the treated group, a difference of 13%. At 28-30 months, the figures were 52% and 40%, respectively, giving a difference of 12%, which is very much the same as for the 16-18 month period. The bottom line was that for every three years treated, one year's disability was saved: other endpoint related to time to need a wheelchair, and MRI data were also positive. Furthermore, the benefit was independent of relapses and baseline disability. Based on these results of this trial a license was issued in Europe for the prescription of interferon ß-1b early in 1999.

It was hoped that further data would lend support to the argument that SPMS is slowed by treatment; however, the recently presented SPECTRIMS study did not provide positive data with respect to the slowing of disability by interferon b-1a in SPMS.[52] This study, the full results of which are still to be published, did demonstrate an effect on relapses, and on MRI activity, confirming previous observations, and after co-variate analysis, there was a borderline effect on disability in the higher dose group, but the essential result was negative as far as disability overall was concerned. This finding, in conjunction with general reservations about the outcome of the trial of interferon ß-1ß, has led to a lack of confidence in the use of the drugs in SPMS in general. A fair summary would seem to be that, at the time of writing, there is enough evidence to support its prescription for this patient group in individuals who are still having frequent relapses, but not for those in whom the clinical course is either purely progressive, or in whom relapses are infrequent or non-disabling.

Many practical issues remain, and the issue of efficacy in non-RRMS has yet to be settled to most clinician's satisfaction. The way forward is unclear, but may lie in the organization of much larger, national or multi-national government sponsored trials, the conduct of which will be a massive undertaking.

11.7 Are there any alternatives to Interferon ß-1a and 1b?

11.7.1 Azathioprine

Many countries in Europe, for example France and Germany, use azathioprine in SPMS to a greater degree than in the UK. This drug suppresses both cell-mediated and humoral immunity relatively safely, and is standard treatment for a number of immune-mediated neurological diseases where a steroid-sparing effect is required. Although individual studies with azathioprine have shown no consistent significant benefit in MS, a meta-analysis of five randomized placebo-controlled trials concluded that it significantly reduces the relapse rate in RR and SPMS, but has only a modest effect on the progression of disability.[48] There is also concern about the risk of long-term azathioprine treatment causing non-Hodgkins lymphoma or other malignancies, though these risks appear to be small. At present azathioprine should be considered for patients with aggressive disease who do not do well on, or cannot have one of the new disease-modifying drugs.

11.7.2 Intravenous immunoglobulin

Intravenous immunoglobulin (IVIg) has, like azathioprine, found a valuable place in the management of a number of important neurological conditions, including the inflammatory polyradiculoneuropathies. So far, experience with IVIg in MS is limited, but it appears to show some promise. There are anecdotal reports of improved recovery from disabling relapses following its use. One study of 150 patients with RRMS treated for two years with monthly infusions of IVIg suggested an improvement in the progression of disability compared with placebo,[49] and another small study reported an effect on MRI and relapses.[50] Further data are required before any firm conclusions can be drawn about the place of IVIg in MS, though a large trial is about to get underway to settle this issue.

Number of relapses	Treated	Placebo
0	34%	27%
1-2	48%	44%
3 or more	18%	29%

Table 11.3 Relapse frequency in the glatiramer acetate trial

EDSS change	Worse	Stable	Improved
Treated	20.8%	56%	24.8%
Placebo	28.8%	54.4%	15.2%

Table 11.4 Percentages of patients with EDSS up to 5.5 whose score worsened, improved or remained stable after treatment (EDSS change unconfirmed)

11.7.3 Glatiramer acetate (formerly Copolymer-1)

Of all agents that have undergone clinical trials in MS apart from interferon ß, to which it is similar in efficacy, glatiramer acetate has shown greatest promise. The drug is administered daily by subcutaneous injection, and is very well tolerated. In well-conducted and properly analyzed placebo-controlled trials of RRMS patients, Glatiramer acetate reduced the relapse frequency, giving an overall reduction in relapse rate of 29% compared to placebo[51], a finding comparable to that with b-interferon (Table 11.3). Furthermore, preliminary five year data suggest that this reduction in relapse rate is maintained, although the results reflect only those patients who were willing to continue on therapy (i.e. those who were obtaining benefit from treatment).

M ULTIPLE SCLEROSIS

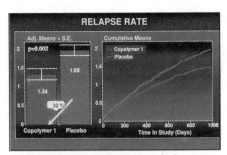

Figure 11.1: MRI confirms a marked reduction in disease activity, which is dose related

It was also claimed that glatiramer acetate had a positive effect on disability measures, though to date, the most rigorous methods of analysis have not been so convincing. A significantly larger proportion of patients on active treatment improved and a smaller one deteriorated (Table 11.4). After three years, a total of 34 of 125 patients improved (compared to 15 of 125 on placebo) by one or more EDSS point, whereas only 23 (compared with 39 on placebo) deteriorated by the same amount, a statistically significant outcome in favor of glatiramer acetate. However, to date, it has not been possible to demonstrate a more robust effect on disability by finding a significantly smaller proportion that do not progress over a defined period of time as was shown, for example, in the second interferon ß-1a study of RRMS patients.

The MRI study showed that there is also a significant positive effect on disease activity as measured by the number of enhancing and new lesions on serial scanning: there was a mean reduction in these parameters of 35%: not as impressive as interferon ß, but still good evidence of efficacy. Overall, the trial results for glatiramer acetate in RRMS are encouraging, and it is hoped that this agent represents a valuable alternative or supplement to interferon ß for these patients, although its exact place in the armamentarium remains to be established (as does its price). Trials of its efficacy in SPMS are also underway.

It is of considerable interest that oral glatiramer is now available and beginning clinical efficacy trials in the US, UK and elsewhere.

11.8 Summary

The last few years have been the most exciting that modern physicians with an interest in MS have experienced. For the first time we have several treatments available which, when used on their own, or perhaps, in the future, in logical combination (what effect interferon ß-1a in combination with Glatiramer acetate?) have demonstrable benefits on the natural history of RR and probably also SPMS. The pharmaceutical industry, has so far largely ignored the most disabling form of MS, namely PPMS, but perhaps this will change. Further advances are on the way, with T-cell vaccination programs and trials of anti-cytokine antibodies well-advanced in planning or actually underway, but so far the 30% reduction in disease activity barrier has not been broken.

For interferon ß there is now evidence that efficacy is dose-related, and the delay in disease progression achieved with interferon ß-1a, 22 and 44 mcg three times weekly, will, if maintained in the long-term, have a considerable impact on the quality of life of individual patients.

We anticipate at every international meeting the results of exciting new trials, some with more hope than others, and several of which are continuing at present. At the recent ECTRIMS 1999, for example, mitoxanthrone became a new contender for the crown of first compound definitely to slow the rate of deterioration in SPMS.

However, one feels that, rather like the difference between learning to swim and deep sea diving, the real breakthrough has not yet been made. Perhaps treatment very early in the course of MS will further improve the efficacy of the existing agents on the disease course, and we await with interest the results of on-going clinical trials.

At present, in the UK at least, the position with respect to interferon b-1a and b has been attempted to be summarized in a recent document issued by the Association of British Neurologists, entitled "Guidelines for the use of beta interferons in multiple sclerosis".[53] In this document, it is stated that for relapsing-remitting disease, candidates for treatment should satisfy the criteria:

1. able to walk 11 yards (approx. 10 meters) with or without assistance (based on the SPMS trial results, NOT the RRMS trials which stipulated 109 yards (approx. 100 meters) without aid or rest);

2. at least two definite relapses in the previous two years;

3. adult age group.

For patients with SPMS, the following comments are offered:

"We cannot unequivocally recommend this treatment at present". However, should beta interferon be considered for patients with SPMS, then:

1. they should be able to walk 11 yards (approx. 10 meters) with or without assistance;

2. there may or may not be superimposed relapses;

Multiple Sclerosis

3. there has been gradually increasing disability for a minimum of six months;

4. the disease is clinically active within the last two years;

5. adult age group.

These proposals, published in June, 1999, did not take into account the SPECTRIMS trial first presented later the same month, and clinicians are now more likely to feel that the comments made above concerning RELAPSE activity are more useful as guidance in patients with SPMS being considered for treatment with beta interferon.

Despite these unequivocal advances, largely brought about by the pharmaceutical industry's development of agents capable of modifying the activity of the disease in the medium term (and in the hope of large returns for their efforts), practicing clinicians who are in daily contact with patients who suffer this disease of unknown cause, and without anything remotely approaching a cure, are well aware that, with limited resources at their disposal, they could still spend their money in a better way than prescribing one of the new drugs applicable to only some of their patients. For the rest, mainly those with more advanced and wholly irreversible disability, there is no realistic hope of a new drug that will make them better; they must rely on the capricious support and resources some have, and some do not. Surely, our energies must not be diverted from the needs of the whole MS population?

Basic science will continue to provide clues to, and advances in, this tantalizing disease, but meanwhile, the clinicians would be very satisfied if their efforts could lead to the provision of proper and properly coordinated support services for all their patients. Therapy centers, nurse specialists, clinics for the newly-diagnosed and other resources are available for a very small proportion of MS sufferers depending on where they live, whereas others have absolutely nothing and no-one to turn to except what they organize themselves. This invidious situation is not easily resolved, but the recently raised profile of the disease, the greater public awareness of its more hopeful side, and above all the gradual but progressive development of specialist therapy groups led by highly trained nurses, are all major steps in the right direction.

It is the opinion of many knowledgeable people that the introduction of new treatments, such as glatiramer acetate, remains a small part of the overall challenge of MS and, while we embark upon the uncertain wait for the cure, we must not lose sight of the needs of most of our patients.

It seems that, rather like antiepileptic drugs, anything you can now think of will reduce relapse rate by 30%. The next step will be far more difficult, to develop a compound which breaks and goes beyond the 50% barrier. That would be the beginning of the end for MS, not just the end of the beginning.

MULTIPLE SCLEROSIS

References

1   Compston DAS. The 150th anniversary of the first depiction of the lesions of multiple sclerosis. *J Neurol Neurosurg Psychiat* 1988; **51**: 1249-1252.

2   Compston DAS. Genetic epidemiology of multiple sclerosis. *J Neurol Neurosurg Psychiat* 1997; **62**: 553-561.

3   Dean G. Annual incidence, prevalence and mortality in white South African-born and in white immigrants to South Africa. *Br Med J* 1967; **2**: 724-730.

4   Fog T., Hyllested K. Prevalence of disseminated sclerosis in the Faroes, the Orkneys, and Shetland. *Acta Neurol Scand* 1966;**42** (suppl 19): 9-11.

5   Robertson NP, Fraser M, Deans J, Clayton D, Compston DAS. Age-adjusted recurrence risks for relatives of patients with multiple sclerosis. *Brain* 1996;**119**: 449-455.

6   McDonald WI, Miller DH and Barnes D. The pathological evolution of multiple sclerosis. *Neuropath Appl Neurobiol* 1992; **18**: 319-334.

7   Poser CM, Paty DW, Scheinberg LC et al. New diagnostic criteria for multiple sclerosis: guidelines for research protocols. *Ann Neurol* 1983; **13**: 227-231.

8   Halliday AM, McDonald WI and Mushin J. Delayed visual evoked response in optic neuritis. *Lancet* 1972; **1**: 982-985.

9   Miller DH, Grossman RI, Reingold SC and McFarlane HF. The role of magnetic resonance techniques in understanding and managing multiple sclerosis. *Brain* 1998; **121**: 3-24

10 Miller DH. MRI safe and sensitive in diagnosing MS. *MRI Decisions* 1988;**2**:17-24.

11 Morrissey SP, Miller DH, Kendall BE et al. The significance of brain magnetic resonance imaging abnormalities at presentation with clinically isolated syndromes suggestive of multiple sclerosis. Brain 1993;**116**: 135-146.

12 O'Riordan JI, Thompson AJ, Kingsley DPE et al. The prognostic value of brain MRI in clinically isolated syndromes of the CNS. *Brain* 1998; **121**: 495-503.

13 Kidd D, Thorpe JW, Thompson AJ, et al. Spinal cord MRI using multi-array coils and fast spin echo. II: findings in multiple sclerosis. *Neurol* 1993; **43**: 2632-2637.

14 Youl BD, Turano G, Miller DH, et al. The pathophysiology of optic neuritis: an association of gadolinium leakage with clinical and electrophysiological deficits. *Brain* 1991; **114**: 2437-2450.

15 Lublin FD and Reingold SC. Defining the clinical course of multiple sclerosis: results of an international survey. *Neurology* 1996; **46**: 907-911.

16 Weinshenker BG, Bass B, Rice GPA, et al. The natural history of multiple sclerosis: A geographically based study. 1. Clinical course and disability. *Brain* 1989; **112**: 133-146

17 Phadke JG. Clinical aspects of multiple sclerosis in north-east Scotland with particular reference to its course and prognosis. *Brain* 1990;**113**: 1597-1628.

18 Kraft GH, Freal JE, Coryell JK, et al. Multiple sclerosis: early prognostic guidelines. *Arch Psy Med Rehabil* 1981;**62**: 54-58.

19 Barnes D, McDonald WI. Ocular manifestations of multiple sclerosis (2) Abnormalities of eye movements. *J Neurol Neurosurg Psychiat* 1992; **55**: 863-868.

20 Betts CD, D'Mellow MT and Fowler CJ. Urinary symptoms and the neurological features of bladder dysfunction in multiple sclerosis. *J Neurol Neurosurg Psychiat* 1993; **56**: 245-250.

21 Archibald CJ, McGrath PJ Ritvo PG et al. Pain prevalence, severity and impact in a clinic sample of multiple sclerosis patients. *Pain* 1994;**58**: 89-93.

22 Fisk JD, Pontefract A Ritvo PJ et al. The inpact of fatigue on patients with multiple sclerosis. *Can J Neurol Sci* (1994); **21**: 9-14

23 Mitchell G. Update on multiple sclerosis therapy. **Med Clin North Am** (1993); **77** (**1**): 231-249

24 Damek DM and Shuster EA. Pregnancy and multiple sclerosis. Mayo Clinic Proc (1997); **72** (**10**): 977-989.

25 Rudick RA. Helping patients live with multiple sclerosis. What primary care physicians can do. *Postgrad Med* (1990); **88**: 197-207.

26 Weinshenker BG. The natural history of multiple sclerosis. *Neurol Clin* (1995); **13**: 119-146.

27 Young RR. Spasticity: a review. *Neurol* (1994); **44 suppl 9**: S12-S20

28 Nguyen JP, Degos DJ. Thalamic stimulation and proximal tremor: a specific target in the ventrointermedius thalami. **Arch Neurol** (1993); **50**: 498-500.

29 Betts CD, Jones SJ, Fowler CG et al. Erectile dysfunction in multiple sclerosis. Associated neurological and neurophysiological deficits, and treatment of the condition. *Brain* (1994); **117**: 1303-1310.

30   Thompson AJ, Kennard C, Swash M et al. Relative efficacy of methylprednisolone and ACTH in the treatment of relapse in multiple sclerosis. *Neurol* (1989); **39**: 969-971.

31   Milligan NM, Newcombe R, Compston DAS. A double-blind controlled trial of high dose methylprednisolone in patients with multiple sclerosis: 1. Clinical effects. *J Neurol Neurosurg Psychiat* (1987); **50**: 511-516.

32   Alam SM, Kyriakides T, Lowden M, Newman PK. Methylprednisolone in multiple sclerosis: a comparison of oral with intravenous therapy at equivalent high dose. *J Neurol Neurosurg Psychiat* (1993); **56**: 1219-1220.

33   Beck RW, Cleary PA, Anderson MM et al. A randomized, controlled trial of corticosteroids in the treatment of acute optic neuritis. *New Engl J Med* 1992; **326 (9)**:581-588.

34   Barnes D, Hughes RAC, Morris RW et al. Randomized trial of oral and intravenous methylprednisolone in acute relapses of multiple sclerosis. *Lancet* (1997); **349**: 902-906.

35   Sellebjerg F, Frederiksen JL, Nielsen PM and Olesen J. Double-blind, randomized, placebo-controlled study of oral, high-dose methylprednisolone in attacks of MS. *Neurol* (1998); **51**: 529-534.

36   The IFNB Multiple Sclerosis Study Group. Interferon beta-1b is effective in relapsing-remitting multiple sclerosis. 1. Clinical results of a multi-center, randomized, double-blind, placebo-controlled trial. *Neurol* (1993); **43**: 655-661.

37   Jacobs LD, Cookfair DL, Rudick RA et al. Intramuscular interferon beta-1a for disease progression in relapsing multiple sclerosis. *Ann Neurol* (1996); **39**: 285-94.

38   Runkel L, Meier W, Pepinsky RB et al. Structural and functional differences between glycosylated and nonglycosylated forms of humen interferon ß. *Pharm Res* (1998); **15**: 641-9.

39   PRISMS (Prevention of Relapses and Disability by Interferon ß-1a Subcutaneously in Multiple Sclerosis) Study Group. Randomized double-blind, placebo-controlled study of interferon beta 1a in relapsing/remitting multiple sclerosis. *Lancet* (1998); **352**: 1498-1504.

40   Trapp BD, Peterson J, Ranshoff RM et al. Axonal transection in the lesions of multiple sclerosis. *New Engl J Med* (1998); *338*: 278-85.

41   US National Multiple Sclerosis Society Disease Management Consensus Statement.

42   Williams GJ, Witt PL. Comparative study of the pharmacodynamic and pharmacologic effects of Betaseron and Avonex. *J Interferon Cytokine Res* (1998); **18**: 967-75.

43   Alam J, McAllister A, Scaramucci J, Jones W, Rogge M. Pharmacokinetics and pharmacodynamics of interferon beta-1a in healthy volunteers after intravenous, subcutaneous or intramuscular administration. (1997) *J Clin Invest*, **14**: 35-43.

44   Munafo A, Trinchard-Lugan I, Nguyen TXQ, Buraglio M. Bioavailability of recombinant human interferon ß-1a after intramuscular and subcutaneous administration. *Eur J Neurol* (1998); **5**: 187-93.

45   Blumhardt LD. Clinical results and outcome measures from the multiple sclerosis PRISMS study. In: Siva A, Kesselring J, Thompson AJ, eds. *Frontiers in Multiple Sclerosis*, volume 2. London, UK: *Martin Dunitz*, 1999; pp217-222.

46   Freedman MS for the OWIMS Study Group. Dose-dependent clinical and magnetic resonance imaging efficacy of IFN ß-1a (Rebif°) in multiple sclerosis. *Ann Neurol* (1998); **44**: 992 (Abstract).

47   European Study Group on Interferon ß-1b in Secondary Progressive MS. Placebo-controlled multicenter randomized trial of interferon ß-1b in treatment of secondary progressive multiple sclerosis. *Lancet* (1998); **352**: 1491-1497.

48   Yudkin PL, Ellison GW, Ghezzi A et al. Overview of azathioprine treatment in multiple sclerosis. *Lancet* (1991); **338**: 1051-55.

49   Fazekas F, Deisenhammer F, Strasser-Fuchs S, Nahler G, Mamoli B, for the Austrian Immunoglobulin in Multiple Sclerosis Study Group. Randomized placebo-controlled trial of monthly intravenous immunoglobulin therapy in relapsing-remitting multiple sclerosis. *Lancet* (1997); **349**: 589-593.

50   Sorensen PS, Wanscher B, Jensen CV et al. Intravenous immunoglobulin G reduces MRI activity in relapsing multiple sclerosis. *Neurology* 1998; **50**: 1273-81.

51   Johnson KP, Brooks BR, Cohen JA et al. Copolymer-1 reduces relapse rate and improved disability in relapsing-remitting multiple sclerosis. Results for a phase III multicenter, double-blind, placebo-controlled trial. *Neurology* (1995); **45**: 1268-76.

52 The SPECTRIMS Study Group. Secondary progressive efficacy clinical trial of recombinant interferon beta-1a in MS. Presented at the European Neurological Society, Milan, Italy. June 1999.

53 Association of British Neurologists. Guidelines for the use of beta interferon in multiple sclerosis. ABN, 27 Boswell Street, London CW1N 3JZ, UK. June 1999.